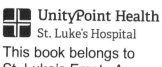
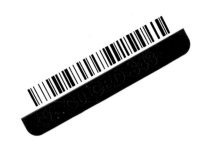
Journeys:

Stories of Pregnancy After Loss

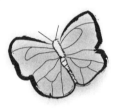

Edited by Amy L. Abbey

Published by WovenWord Press
811 Mapleton Ave.
Boulder, CO 80304
www.wovenword.com

Cover design © 2006 by Jeanine Davis
Book design © 2006 by Vicki McVey
Author photo © 2006 by Anna Orologlio

ISBN 0-9766678-3-5
ISBN13 978-0-9766678-3-4
LCCN 2006921657

1. Pregnancy & childbirth 2. Grief 3. Healing
4. Subsequent pregnancy

To all our children

ACKNOWLEDGEMENTS

Writing this book has been a wonderful journey. First and foremost I need to thank my fellow writers: Michele Carey-Moody, Nancy Annett, Eric Abbey, Rosanna Tarrega, Lynn McGinnis, Patty Bradley, Lynn Vernillo, Linda Marie Vosseller, Cindy Canny and Donna DeAngelis, and their families. They put up with a myriad of email notes, revision suggestions and just plain old pestering by me to get their stories written. I would have no book without them.

Next I would like to thank Sheila Dierks at WovenWord Press who initially intercepted my email synopsis and whose interest in this project was piqued.

The authors and I wish to express deep gratitude to Margaret Fusco, Anna Orologio, Monica Wakely and Martha Weiss, who led all of us through the path of our grief, never doubting for a moment we could and would go on with our lives. Their commitment to us, individually and collectively, enabled us to live again, to find our new normals. We are all grateful.

I wish to thank my family and friends, the ones who "get it" and the ones who don't. It is probably the ones who don't get it I held in my heart as I was preparing this. An extra special thank you to Alex, who pulled me out of some of my darkest moments.

I would not have my children if it weren't for the expert medical care I received from Dr. David Eysler and his compassionate staff. And for their numerous prayers for me when I could not pray myself, many thanks to Trina Vicks, Jody Steinhardt and posthumously Terry Salvaggio.

A heartfelt appreciation goes out to Cary Kappel and Joshua G. Fensterstock, who advised me on some of the legal aspects of creating this book.

For her dazzling artistic skills and wonderful friendship, a hug of thanks goes to Jeanine Davis.

For finding me and offering a kernel of hope, and for her continued diligence to keep me focused on the future, a thank you is offered to Stephanie C. Gross.

My children Alison and Adam; I look at them in wonder every day. They are here because others are not and have enriched my life so much; I can't imagine a life without them. They have endured more Barney and Sesame Street than I would ever have wanted, while I worked on this manuscript.

Lastly, there is my husband Eric to thank. He never gave up on me and many times I never understood why. I guess that is what marriage is all about.

INTRODUCTION

If you are reading this book, then you or someone you love has had a pregnancy loss and may even be pregnant again. It is my hope that you find some kernel of connection and encouragement here. Parents who share your experiences composed all the stories. We aren't writers or medical professionals by a long shot. Many of the stories are written in a "stream of consciousness" fashion: we just sat at our keyboards and typed from our hearts what we remembered about our experiences. Sometimes our voices are desperate, sometimes we are unsure, and sometimes we are just sad. There are similarities and differences in all the tales. We come from different backgrounds yet were all forced to join a club we didn't want to belong to. And yet in joining the club and taking the steps to heal, we hope others will find the strength to do what we have done.

The book started slowly. I grieved for months after losing my son Solomon, and I found limited help in the "outside world." For every one person's kind and comforting words, I was met ten-fold with remarks like, "You can have another," or "When you get pregnant again you will forget all about this." And I wondered, how do you forget a life that was inside of you? I would explain over and over again to my husband that I felt people were treating me as if I'd lost my car keys, and I couldn't understand why so many "outsiders" did not understand my grief.

I started journaling when I came home from the hospital empty-armed. After I had my second loss and D&C, I outlined a book to write. And after I had my two children, I modified my outline drastically and came up with the idea of women sharing their stories, instead of just me sharing mine. This book covers stories from parents who have had first trimester miscarriages, second trimester deliveries, full-term stillbirths and infant death.

Each parent authored two stories: the loss and the subsequent pregnancy. Our stories are all different yet our grief is the same.

During my grief, I sought support in so many places: my family, friends, books, the Internet and professionals. I oftentimes felt like a patchwork quilt that was slowly being assembled, never really knowing what the finished product would be, or who I would be once I was "whole" again. I learned quickly that most people offer little if they have not experienced this themselves. But I also learned that sometimes loss is loss, and I did find comfort in unusual places. There were times I just blurted out my sadness to whoever was there as it was impossible to keep my feelings bottled up. I never knew at any given moment when the grief would overcome me. In doing so I made connections with many wonderful women and men, most of whom I would never had known otherwise. I was always astonished to hear another family's loss story. I had such a naivety that pregnancy loss was an everyday occurrence. And I tried to figure out what kept me marching forward.

At this book's printing it will be six years since Solomon and his little brother passed through my life. Am I "over it?" Not really. It isn't something to get over. Have I integrated my experience into my life? I think I have. I was told to expect at least a year of heartache, realizing the milestones my children would not have: holidays like Mother's Day and "firsts," like smiles. But there are other milestones.

Many of my friends' children started Kindergarten and I was saddened Solomon wouldn't. At my fortieth birthday, watching Alison and Adam running around, I realized someone was missing. I know now his loss will be faced repeatedly through the years, not just on his anniversary.

I was asked by an acquaintance recently, how long was it until I felt comfortable to really move forward. For me it was four years since the losses. I remember distinctly it was around the time of my son Adam's second birthday that I realized I could exhale.

I still miss my children and recognize the importance of their existence. From conception they were gifts I wanted very much. But unbeknownst to me, they would be gifts I would never receive. They cleared the path for Alison and Adam, the gifts that were waiting.

I hope you will read this book and seek comfort in knowing you are not alone. The resources at the end I hope will serve as a guide if you want more information.

Peace on your journey.

Amy L. Abbey

FOREWORD

Façade

Love insists our hope
Hidden in winter's façade.
A child. An image.
A memory. A promise.
Yet,
We shall unveil its wonder;
…The gift of tomorrow,
And why we love, today.©

Michael R. Berman, M. D.

When a child dies before or after birth, parents experience the "the saddest of sadness," often bearing profound grief, unremitting guilt and a sense of hopelessness that endures despite efforts by friends, family, counselors and physicians. For all birth orders, but most pronounced for those having first children, the parent's loss is accompanied by a very real and haunting fear that they will be childless and without a natural family. Despite the best intentions and compassion by their doctors, statistics and examples, they mourn, absent of hope.

In this remarkable book, Amy Abbey and all the parents have bonded the ephemeral hopelessness and forsaken dreams of parents' lost children with inherent passions and determinations central to all humankind. With example after example, all the authors have shone light on the darkness of despairing families. Here, hope surfaces from the depths of lifeless dreams. The reader becomes transported and transformed, renewed and refreshed.

The words and stories and thoughts which follow emanate our pleas of why we must allow hope to be imperishable and "why we love," prevail.

Michael R. Berman, M. D.
Clinical Professor of Obstetrics, Gynecology and Reproductive Sciences
Yale University School of Medicine
Founder and President
Hygeia Foundation, Inc. and Institute for Perinatal Loss & Bereavement

Where Am I In The Journey?

By Anna Orologio, LMSW

Everything has a beginning, middle, and end,
But where am I in the journey?
For some, the beginning is the end,
For others, the end is the beginning,
But where am I in the journey?
Each thing we learn, each thing we experience,
Fills our well, a well in need of filling.
But where am I in the journey?
We all have tasks that we must master
Like the points on a clock,
But where am I in the journey?
We each have a path that we
Must follow,
Once complete, we are set free,
But where am I in the journey?
Oh, but to have that answer…
The journey is what we make it…

Disclaimer

The stories contained in this book are the authors' recollections and retelling of their experiences from pregnancy loss through subsequent pregnancy. This book is not intended nor is it implied to be a substitute for professional medical advice, and any medical information contained in this book is not intended to be diagnostic or treatment in any way. *The authors are not medical professionals.*

The authors do not recommend using any specific books, videotapes, the Internet or other educational media as the sole information-gathering tool. As medical information can change rapidly, you are strongly encouraged to discuss all health matters and concerns with your physician before embarking on new diagnostic or treatment strategies.

The names of the hospitals are included for reference only and in no way are intended to be a reflection of the hospitals' care. The names of the doctors have been intentionally omitted for their protection.

MICHELE

My Two Unnamed Angels

A person's a person, no matter how small
Horton Hears a Who! Dr. Seuss

Our story began during the summer of 2001. Tom and I were married for two and half years. After lots of discussion and planning we decided to begin trying to have a baby. We did all of the correct procedures: finding a doctor with a good reputation, affiliated with a hospital where we wanted to deliver.

I began an exercise program and started charting my cycle. The doctor and I discussed prenatal planning, took notes and determined what tests would be necessary since I was soon to turn thirty four. Now off the pill, I began modifying my diet. We picked up an ovulation kit and our first fertile time according to the test results was September 11. We live on Long Island and my husband works in midtown Manhattan near the United Nations building.

September 11 was a terrible day for us. The last time I spoke to Tom was at ten A.M., after the towers had been struck but before they collapsed. Tom told me he and his brother were going to try to walk out of Manhattan. I didn't hear again from him until four thirty P.M. There was no part of our lives unaffected by the losses. We lost friends, family and neighbors and our sense of security.

We knew there would be an opportunity to try again the next month, but now we needed to focus our attention on memorial services and taking care of our family and friends. Tom began to have nightmares from what he saw that day and I didn't want to push him. I knew I was in a stressful environment that would only complicate trying to conceive. We decided to take care of our family and friends and to help our community heal. Short-term that allowed us to heal ourselves as well.

After months of trying, we finally got pregnant at the end of May 2002. We seemed to be going on our merry way when I started spotting June 26. I was only six weeks pregnant and I still hadn't even been to the doctor. My first prenatal appointment wasn't for another two weeks. I was at work and phoned my new doctor and found out she was on maternity leave. Staff told me to come in anyway.

I called Tom; he told me not to worry, it was probably just routine.

I was scared. The waiting room was filled with expectant mothers. I needed to use the ladies' room. I was bleeding much more now and I knew it wasn't good. I ended up miscarrying in the waiting room. There was nothing anyone could do. The sonogram technician stated there was nothing there, the sac and everything was gone. I asked her for a sanitary napkin since I was still bleeding so heavily. I felt terrible; I just cried and cried. The nursing staff was really wonderful but they didn't want me back in the main waiting area.

They put me in an office. It began to rain and there was a lot of thunder and lightning, then it really poured. The rain was coming down so hard it was drowning out my sobs. I was trying to hold them in so I didn't scare any of the other patients.

A nurse asked me if I wanted to call anyone and I realized there was no one. Tom was on a train heading to our home and we didn't have cell phones yet. As I sat there I heard an odd sound in the examining rooms around me, a whooshing sound. I didn't know at the time it was the fetal heart monitor and that was a little blessing. I think if I'd known it at the time it would have been unbearable.

The covering doctor came into the office and told me he was so sorry for my loss but he would need to examine me. This was the worst exam I'd ever had. He explained the miscarriage was complete and he couldn't have stopped it. He drew blood for testing and suggested I have a follow up appointment in two weeks.

I was on my way out of the office when one of the nurses gently touched my arm. I completely lost it. I started crying uncontrollably. She took me into the little area behind the glass and asked me if I wanted a glass of water. I just shook my head. I couldn't even speak. Then she asked me if I was all right to drive and I said I would be OK.

I drove home in a daze. As I walked into my house Tom asked how it had gone. I collapsed sobbing and he picked me up, kissed my hairline and said he was so sorry.

During my checkup two weeks later the doctor, a different member of the practice, said my progesterone level was low, a possible reason for the miscarriage. She mentioned next time she would suggest progesterone suppositories to help raise my levels. She said there were no guarantees the suppositories even worked but they also didn't hurt anything. I didn't like this as an answer so I went back to my old doctor in Manhattan whom I'd left due to distance, but for my peace of mind I did it.

After reviewing my chart, my doctor suggested a procedure to make sure I didn't have risk factors for ectopic pregnancy. I had an infection and a procedure several years prior and was possibly predisposed.

Emotionally this was a difficult time. We hadn't told anyone of our loss. Ironically my parents had had four losses due to the Rh-negative factors. I know it would seem logical to call my Dad and discuss our situation but I just couldn't. He is a wonderful man but he would relive his losses and I just couldn't bear to hear about them.

Tom and I felt we should do the procedure and begin again. I think in certain ways it hadn't been real to him. At the end of July my sister-in-law told everyone she was expecting. I was happy for them but crushed for myself. This would be her second child and I was trying so hard just to have my first. As I wrestled with these feelings, of which I was totally ashamed, we received a call from my in-laws; my sister-in-law was having a miscarriage and she didn't want anyone to call. I totally understood and very gently several weeks later confided to her we, too, had a loss and understood what they were going through. We just asked they not share this information with anyone and she told me how she had wished she hadn't announced their pregnancy.

At the end of August 2002, I had a hysterosalpingogram, to make sure my tubes were clear and there were no blockages or cysts to worry about. After the procedure I was sore and cramped for a few days. Additionally, I had blood drawn to make sure there were no infections. All of my tests came back normal.

We were allowed to begin trying again. Back to the store I went to purchase more ovulation kits and to start charting for the most fertile time.

In October I was told my job would be eliminated. Tom and I discussed perhaps it was a good thing and I could start to look for a less stressful job.

It seemed everywhere I looked everyone was pregnant, which was difficult, but I just kept telling myself I was going to be able to get pregnant and it was just bad luck with the first loss and to get over it.

In November I found out I was pregnant. I called my OB's office, told them I was pregnant and reminded them I had a previous early miscarriage. I began taking progesterone suppositories. During the first week of December I started cramping, I was eight weeks pregnant. I was sent for a sonogram. On December 6, my OB called to tell me they thought I had a molar pregnancy. We would wait to see if I began to miscarry. If I didn't, the doctor would do a D&C, a procedure to scrape the inside of the uterus of all contents. If it were a molar pregnancy, I would need treatment and have to delay trying to conceive another baby for another year.

I was crushed. I didn't know this was possible but as I read on the websites my doctor suggested I learned more. I kept thinking, *What are the odds? A miscarriage with my first pregnancy and now with my second some rare type of pregnancy that isn't even a pregnancy?* The odds, even on the websites, were stated as so small of getting this type of complication. To put the two losses together with one person was astounding.

In an even more cruel twist of fate I'd agreed to co-host a party at my house that night and there were fifteen women coming to my house. I had no way of calling off the party.

I had just started spotting. I didn't even have time to call Tom. I picked my sister-in-law up and told her the news. "I'm pregnant but it isn't going well. I'm losing another pregnancy." I handed her the printout from my OB, "Please read this. It will explain better then I can."

She promised to help make the party move along and not let any of the guests stay too long. I went home and handed my husband the printout about molar pregnancies and then the doorbell rang. I had to go and entertain my guests. I put on a happy face; the party ended around eleven thirty P.M. and the guests went home.

The reality of my situation hit and I sobbed. As directed I called the doctor's office in the morning and the covering doctor answered. He was wonderful. As the weekend progressed I spoke to this doctor seven times. I was having a miscarriage and losing another child.

The holiday season is often difficult for many people but going through a loss during this time is excruciating. I remember watching the lighting of the Rockefeller Center Christmas Tree on TV and praying to God, "Please don't let this happen again." At times I wanted them to do a D&C so it would be over but the doctor warned me it could put me at risk for Asherman's Syndrome (adhesions in the uterus) which would give me conception troubles in the future. So I continued to suffer silently. It took a total of three weeks for the miscarriage to be complete. Thankfully, it was not a molar pregnancy.

My company told me they had another position for me. Small consolation, but I thought it might give me something to focus on.

As the weeks grew on, I realized I couldn't stop crying and the depression was getting worse, so I asked for medication. I started Prozac and began to feel less crazy. I knew I needed more help and I sought out a grief group. I was lucky enough to find one specializing in prenatal bereavement at the hospital my doctor's office is affiliated with.

I started going to my group in January 2003. Tom didn't want to go. He is a private person and deals with things differently but he supported me any way he could.

In this group there were five of us: two couples and me. One couple had lost their son at sixteen weeks. The other couple had several losses, a daughter at twenty eight weeks, an early miscarriage and most recently another daughter at eighteen weeks. We met for six weeks with a social worker and it really helped to give me closure.

I urge anyone who has had a loss to do this because it truly helps you mourn. Although the other couples had later term losses I still felt it was important for me to recognize my lost children and mourn their deaths. I never had a picture or even a sonogram photo. I never held them or had a name for them but I know my two unnamed angels are in heaven looking down on my husband and me.

So as a fresh start Tom and I took a small vacation, a long weekend to the Berkshires Mountains. This was for Presidents' Weekend. We went hiking with llamas and antiquing and said goodbye to our lost children and hello to the possibilities of a new future.

Hiking with the llamas was a unique and magical experience. They are such majestic animals and incredibly gentle. It was a bitter cold day in February 2003. There was snow on the ground and we hiked on the snow mobile trails. It was a great way to shut out all of the noise and stress of our lives. Tom and I loved this experience. He was a little hesitant about hiking with llamas but in the end I know he enjoyed it just as much as I did. We spent this weekend discussing whether we wanted to really try and get pregnant another time. Many of our older relatives said, "You are young and this was just a blip on the radar. Try again and you will get over it." I knew having been involved with a prenatal bereavement group this was a normal reaction from people who just didn't understand this kind of loss.

Many holidays and anniversaries have come and gone since the losses: the first Mother's Day, the due dates and year anniversaries. Throughout all of those milestones I've felt sorrow, and the grief has come back. I like to think of it when I describe it as ocean waves; the feelings come and they go but you never forget. It does get easier because, like beach glass the rough edges of your grief are worn down, but in the end you still have this gem, this beach glass, the memory of your lost children.

My story is dedicated to all of you who have had first trimester losses. There is very little reading for you and you feel as if your loss isn't as important as later term losses. That isn't the case. Every loss is painful, personal and important.

The Magic of the Llamas - Delaney Bridget

My mama is a llama.
Is Your Mama a Llama? Deborah Guarino

Tom and I found out I was pregnant in March. I was absolutely overjoyed and terrified at the exact same time. I called my doctor and asked for progesterone suppositories. When I went in the same nurses who helped me through my losses were there and they were so incredibly gentle with me.

I was still pretty fragile. Sylvia was the nurse and she took me on as her special patient. Since I'd lost both pregnancies in the early first trimester, the doctors wanted to closely monitor my HGC and progesterone levels, the "pregnancy" hormones. Previously they were low, so this time I was taking progesterone suppositories twice a day.

I was also on a low version of Prozac. The doctors didn't want me to come off too soon; which was fine with Tom and me. The only time it would be a problem is if I wanted to nurse. *Let me take one step at a time,* I thought.

I went three times a week to have my blood drawn and I tracked everything. I held my breath every time I called the office. It takes a whole day to get the results. I prayed before I picked up the phone and dialed.

I already told Tom I didn't want to tell anyone I was pregnant until I was sure it was OK. He agreed and we kept silent.

My first appointment was at the end of April. Tom came with me. I was so excited to be able to even have an appointment. We went for the sonogram and there it was, a baby. I was so amazed. Finally a picture of my child. I was so excited. I thought this was definitely a sign of good things to come.

I kept getting my blood drawn twice a week. The HCG (Human Chorionic Gonadotropin, also known as the pregnancy hormone) numbers kept growing and it was wonderful. At eight and a half weeks I started spotting and I began freaking out. I called my doctor and they told me to come right in. They also instructed me to be on bed-rest for a few days. I was already seeing my doctors once a week and I began to feel better.

I went to my boss and explained I would need to work from home. The spotting stopped and I realized I needed to take it easy. I was restricted from exercise and told not to lift heavy objects. I was also told no sexual activity. That was OK with me, as I didn't want to do anything to risk this pregnancy.

I also had joined a SPALS support group (this is a Subsequent Pregnancy After Loss group). Led by a rotating group of social workers specializing in prenatal loss, it met every other week. There were moms alone and couples, all who had experienced a pregnancy loss. I joined when I was six weeks along and I truly feel it helped me through what was the most difficult part of my previous pregnancies. I had no idea how much I would need and come to love this group of parents until later.

I finally made it through the first trimester and at another sonogram the doctor noticed I had a low-lying placenta. I was just delighted I had enough progesterone to get a placenta; I didn't care if it was low or high. I just knew I had a baby and placenta to nourish this child. As the doctor explained, this was an issue for delivery later on but not to worry right now. He was concerned the placenta would cover the cervix and prevent a vaginal delivery. I just tried to push this information out of my head and relax and hold on to my baby.

The doctor finally said it would be all right to tell people about our pregnancy. On Mother's Day weekend I went to my mom's house and we told my family I was expecting. We showed them the baby's sonogram pictures in a photo album. The following weekend we told Tom's family. I was a nervous wreck and I kept thinking, *OK, we just told people. Now what's going to happen?* My sister-in-law again was also pregnant. This was a true blessing since she knew what I was going through and was able to help me keep my sanity. We also share the same doctor's office. It made it easier; we could talk about the bedside manner of the different doctors and staff. I know it sounds crazy but it really helped when making appointments. When you go to the doctor's office, with several members, (mine has six doctors), you need to rotate through the entire staff. This way, at delivery, you aren't meeting the doctor-on-call for the very first time.

The next hurdle was the genetic testing. What type of testing did I want? One choice was a blood test called a triple test, also known as an Alpha Feta Protein. Since I was thirty five years old, Down syndrome was a possibility. With a false negative test I would then have to do the amniocentesis anyway. I didn't want to stress myself out and I really wanted one hundred percent accuracy.

We had our amniocentesis scheduled for fifteen weeks.

The test can be frightening and there is also a chance of causing miscarriage. I decided not to watch the insertion of the needle directly but rather indirectly on the sonogram monitor. They need to have the sonogram on you so the doctor doesn't hit the baby with the needle. I kept telling them do whatever they needed to me but don't hurt the baby. I lay very still and I held my breath and the baby wasn't touched. Tom was with me and he didn't do as well. He needed to sit down after seeing the needle. I figured then I had a few months to prep him for the delivery room and I really needed the laughter from the paleness of his face.

Waiting for the results of the amniocentesis was tough. I had an appointment at nineteen weeks to get the results and to have a checkup. The nurse told me the lab needed to rerun the results; they wouldn't be ready then. The doctor came in and I started to cry. I was so worried about the results and the doctor told me it was normal to double-check the results. He gave me another sonogram to show me my baby was fine.

His only concern was my placenta was still low-lying but that could change in the next few months; as the uterus grew the placenta would move upwards. He told me I had an anterior placenta, attached on the front wall of the uterus, not the back, thereby cushioning the movement of the baby. I might not feel the baby move that much. For someone who had previous losses this was disturbing to me but I discussed my concerns with my SPALS group and they helped me settle down.

At twenty two weeks I would get my level II sonogram, at which there is a real up close look at the baby and we could even discover the gender. Tom and I chose not to find out.

Everything at the level II went according to plan except my placenta was still a little low. Oddly I had the same radiologist as in the last pregnancy. He was pretty insensitive because he kept asking questions about the loss. All I'd wanted all along was for a normal pregnancy but after you have had losses there is no such thing.

This was a crazy time emotionally for me. Other people I knew became pregnant and hadn't had previous losses and were, in my eyes, more reckless. My doctors had told me no alcohol or cold cuts in addition to no raw meats. My newly blissful pregnant friends were munching happily along on salami sandwiches and having the occasional glass of wine. There was one friend in particular who hurt me terribly with her insensitivity and she had in fact, known about my losses. She stated to me she could eat and drink whatever she wanted, cold cuts and wine and all, since her progesterone levels were so much higher then mine were. I thought, *Like one thing had to do with another*! This comment made me pull away from her and to this day we aren't as close. I wanted to preserve the memory of my lost children and protect my unborn child from any harsh comments, so I pulled away from her. My SPALS group gave me a lot of comfort during this time. They helped to give me the strength to separate.

I have one very close friend who lives out of state and she was wonderful. When I was feeling bad or overwhelmed I would phone. She would be mad *for me* so I wouldn't stress out and hurt the baby. I love this friend so much; she always had me laughing at the end of a conversation. Without her I couldn't have gotten off the Prozac, as I knew I had to do. She helped me keep things in perspective.

At twenty six weeks I went for glucose testing. I failed miserably. The levels were supposed to be lower than 140 and I was at 199. I went for the three-hour test and I scored the same. I wasn't feeling well. I was very swollen and had gained a lot of weight. I had gestational diabetes. The big fear here is the baby can get too big or develop various health problems. The doctors predicted I could have upwards of a ten-pound-baby.

I was sent to a nutritionist in order to use diet to control the diabetes. I had to test my blood eight to ten times a day. I needed to prick my finger since gestational diabetes needs to be accurate. For anyone who has diabetes and needs to work with their hands I admire them. It hurts more then anyone tells you, not because you do it once but because after time your fingers ache and you try and find an area not as sensitive to prick for the next blood draw.

There was a very strict diet and that wasn't fun. I watched everything I ate. I also had to test my urine so I ate enough and didn't get ketones in my urine. The ketones were very dangerous for the baby.

By the time I was thirty weeks the restricted diet wasn't working. I started going to a perinatologist who specializes in gestational diabetes. They instructed me on how to inject myself with insulin once a day.

I learned our baby would be taken to the Neonatal Intensive Care Unit (NICU) after it was born and tested for glucose levels. By thirty two weeks I had to get special sonograms to check for negative effects from the insulin and be on a baby heart monitor to measure movement. At these visits they also started measuring my blood pressure because of concerns about toxemia.

During this time I'd been practicing something my SPALS friends had mentioned: wearing red on your person brings good luck. So I continued to have my toenails painted red.

We also had a conference in October called Remembrance Day for our lost children. When the idea of a quilt was presented, I decided to participate. I wanted to tie my quilt square to my unborn child so I used the same color paint for my quilt square I used in the nursery Tom and I were setting up.

My quilt square was very plain, just two stencils of an angel with the simple handwritten dates of their losses. In many ways this helped me prepare for the impending arrival of this child because I felt I'd finally preserved, permanently, memory of my lost children.

I was thirty five weeks along and seeing the perinatologist twice a week and my regular OB once a week. My insulin was increased since the diabetes had gotten worse. I was really leaning on the SPALS group during this time.

I was scared. In certain ways I wanted to be induced at this point and save my baby and in other ways I wanted to stay pregnant since I didn't know if the baby's lungs were developed enough. In week thirty six, at the baby measurement sonogram they told us the insulin was doing the job and keeping the baby from getting too big, and the baby was on track developmentally. They estimated it weighed almost six pounds.

By thirty eight weeks my insulin was increased again to larger doses and increased frequency. My thighs were black and blue since the only location you can insert the needles for effectiveness is in the upper legs or the belly, (the belly was out as a location). I asked my doctors to please let it be over. My whole body was swollen, my hands ached from the blood testing and my thighs ached from the needles. They decided to induce.

I was scheduled for Monday, November 10, the first day of my thirty-ninth week. I was so excited. We went to the hospital at seven thirty A.M. and an hour later I was on Pitocin to start contractions. My placenta had moved up and I anticipated a natural delivery. I arrived at the hospital at almost two centimeters dilated.

I thought by the afternoon we would be parents. The nurses cautioned if I had the epidural before I reached four centimeter there was a chance I would backtrack. My contractions had been one on top of another and it was tough since my body was already weakened. At seven P.M. I hadn't progressed and my doctors decided to do a C-section. We didn't get into an operating room until nine P.M. After all the prep we were ready. At nine thirty-three P.M. my daughter Delaney Bridget was born at six pounds fifteen ounces and twenty one inches long. The NICU doctors were there and they took my daughter away.

I wasn't in great shape; I'd started to tremor on the operating table so the entire upper half of my body was shaking. The doctor ordered Demerol to quiet the tremors.

The entire mood of the operating room changed and I knew something was wrong. I could see there was an entire new team of people in the room and I had two of the doctors from my practice working on me. I was bleeding out. I had a condition called placenta accreta; the placenta had grown into the walls of my uterus. The normal procedure is to do a hysterectomy. I joked with the staff and said I wanted to leave with all my parts and they told me they were trying to make that happen. My doctors did some very fancy stitch work and were able to save my uterus.

I left the operating room at eleven forty-five P.M. I was scared and still trembling. They put a special blanket on me and told me I would be in recovery for a while. I wanted to see my new baby and they said I could later. I sent Tom home to rest and call the grandparents.

At three thirty A.M. I spiked a very high fever and the doctors came to my side. Soon after, the nurses brought my daughter to me. I was so excited to see her but I'd been ordered to lie completely flat and I couldn't even lift my arms to hold her.

I was exhausted. As I started to heal the doctors informed me it wasn't certain the stitches would hold and they might have to remove my uterus. I thought about my lost children and my new child and the possibility of never having additional children and the thoughts overwhelmed me.

The stitches healed and held and I still have my uterus today. The prognosis is the next pregnancy will probably be my last because the reoccurrence of the placenta accreta greatly increases after the first time.

Ten months have passed and Tom and I have absolutely enjoyed our beautiful daughter. We have gone back to the Berkshire Mountains and hiked with the llamas, this time with our daughter. Delaney loved these beautiful animals and it was just as magical. It started to rain a bit as we walked through the forest with these beautiful majestic animals and I thought again of our lost children and this was the sign they were happy.

In a certain way it was the circle of grief and happiness coming together. It was truly the circle of life in an emotional sense. Who knows whether or not Delaney will have any siblings or what the possibilities of time will bring. Whatever life presents to us, I know we will be ready. I enjoy every second of Delaney and know whatever happens she will always have two guardian angels to watch over her.

NANCY

Meeting Matthew

From this day on, now and forever you'll be in my heart
No matter what they say, you'll be in my heart always
"You'll Be In My Heart" written by Phil Collins

Where do I begin? Jeff and I always knew we wanted a family from our dating years to the day when we said, "I do." On our fifth wedding anniversary we said this would be the year to start our family. We felt we were stable in our home, careers and finances. Months of trying to conceive passed and nothing happened.

I was charting basal temperatures, I had normal menstrual cycles. I was thirty two years old and Jeff was thirty six. Were we really trying, or was it just words? I think we were just scared we wouldn't be good parents.

Finally we had a positive pregnancy test in May 1997, six months since our anniversary. We couldn't believe we finally got two lines on the test. We were worried Jeff may have been sterile since he had chickenpox in his twenties. There was always that thought, but we never discussed it. So he was ecstatic his "boys could swim." I went to the obstetrician in June for my first prenatal visit. We spoke at length; he took a history and finally did the sonogram. The technician asked me my last menstrual period (LMP) date since we were trying to get pregnant and I gave her the date. She asked me if I was sure. I started doubting myself. I said, "Do you see a heartbeat?" She said, "No, but you may be early because we have a gestational sac on the screen." So, of course, I assumed I got my dates wrong. I was told to come back in two weeks.

Those two weeks felt like an eternity. I got pulled over by a police officer for speeding in a work zone; I was just in a cloud. I was reading *What To Expect When You're Expecting*. I would feel my breasts to see if they were enlarging and firm. Two weeks came and this sonogram showed no heartbeat, just an empty sac. The doctor said it could be a blighted ovum. I dropped the egg but there was no fertilization.

Now the doctor had me go for serial HCGs to see if my hormone levels were going up, thus indicating a viable pregnancy. This meant having blood-work done everyday.

The spotting started and I went for another sonogram, and still an empty sac. Finally the senior OB in the group said, "It looks as if you will abort." I said, "Listen, I'm a physician. Is this a blighted ovum?" He said, "Possibly." He still didn't want to commit.

July 5th I awoke to bright red blood and I knew. It was a holiday weekend. I called the service of my OB/Gyn group, told what was happening and that I was a physician. I was to call the office on Monday to have a follow-up sonogram to make sure there were no remnants left. What a weekend! No one knew I was pregnant except Jeff. I called work, told them I had a virus. I went back after three days, they said, "You look so pale." If they only knew. Three days prior I had gone to the OB, had a sonogram; all was gone. I didn't need a D&C.

Six months later and it was a new year. I made an appointment with another group of OB/Gyns in Garden City after quizzing colleagues about whom they would recommend.

I was impressed. An hour consultation: the OB asked me for a detailed family history, if Jeff worked in a heated environment that can cause a low sperm count or sterility. When he was younger he worked in a pizza place by hot stoves. I felt the questioning was of vital importance. No other doctor asked that before. I was assured at least I knew I was fertile; it's common for first pregnancies to be blighted.

I felt so comfortable. I had a thorough physical exam and was given prenatal vitamins and a prescription for a sperm count for Jeff, to check motility, quality and quantity of the sperm. Jeff did the test and he was fine. He was concerned he was the reason for us not getting pregnant.

As for me, we needed a repeat Pap test due to a lack of endocervical cells, making the pap exam inadequate for evaluation. I made the appointment, had the repeat pap and all was well. The doctor said, "The next time I'll see you is June or sooner if you are pregnant."

By the end of March we had a positive pregnancy test. This time we didn't want to get too excited because of what had happened earlier. Eight weeks later Jeff and I were at the OB together. The doctor asked for the last menstrual period.

Now, to the sonogram. He knew we were nervous and there it was: a sac with a heartbeat. I must have asked several times, "Are you sure?" We started to cry, it finally happened.

I was going for monthly appointments, all was well. At three months we finally told our family and friends. We felt we were safe and out of our first trimester.

At fifteen weeks I started spotting. I was at work and went at night to the OB. They did a sonogram, the heartbeat was there. It was just a low-lying placenta. So I couldn't lift anything, or have intercourse and I had to take it easy until the placenta moved up at around twenty weeks.

A few weeks went by. I woke one Saturday morning to bright red blood and lost my mind. Jeff was home; I was crying, "How could this be happening again?" We went immediately to the OB's office.

The sonogram showed a heartbeat. They reassured me about the low-lying placenta and suggested I take a few days off from work and follow up in a week.

At this time, I only wore white underwear. I wanted to make sure I wouldn't miss anything. I would check myself for spotting in the bathroom hourly. I just couldn't relax. My co-workers knew I was pregnant and could see the stress and worry.

I went to the OB alone on a Saturday feeling great. I met a different OB in the group. I had come for my Alpha-Feto Protein test which can detect neural tube defects and other abnormalities such as Down syndrome, and reported that a week ago I had had bright red blood. He did a sonogram which showed the heartbeat was fine, the placenta moving up. But the cervix looked short and also felt short on palpation. Not knowing if this was normal for me, he wanted me to go to Winthrop University Hospital since the doctor who had seen me prior to pregnancy was on-call there.

I called Jeff. I was doing okay, only going to WUH for a second opinion. I went to the admitting office alone, gave all my information, went up to the floor, and was met by a nurse who gave me a gown. I couldn't believe where I was: in a hospital as a patient. Usually I'm taking care of patients.

My OB arrived with a resident and a bedside sonogram machine. Here we go again. He felt my cervix was slightly shortened and wanted to put in a cerclage (a stitch to keep the cervix closed). It was a precaution and as I am a physician they were even more cautious. I called Jeff and gave him the update. At six P.M. I was going to the operating room. Jeff came to the hospital. When I saw him I started to cry. I was so vulnerable. This was the first time I would spend the night in the hospital as a patient. That was hard for me, to be taken care of by others.

Time went by. I was starving. I went to the OR at eleven P.M. since they had so many emergencies. With spinal anesthesia I was awake but numb from the waist down. All went well. I went to Recovery afterwards for about thirty minutes. I became so nauseated from the anesthesia and from not eating I started vomiting. Now I was being a patient who gave more work to the nurse; what I didn't want in the first place. I was given crackers and started feeling much better.

Next morning I was fine. No one knew I had the cerclage. I didn't want people worrying about me.

Back to work Monday. I was going to the OB every two weeks. After the cerclage, no spotting, all was well. At thirty six weeks they took out the stitch and two weeks later our daughter was born. A perfect baby! Miracles do happen.

When we celebrated Elise's first birthday we began planning to have a sibling for her. The New Year came, 2001.

I made my post-partum appointment with the OB. All was well. He said, "I'll see you in six months or sooner if you get pregnant." Three months passed and we were pregnant.

At my eight-week prenatal visit I told the OB, "After I saw you, within three months I become pregnant." Jokingly he said, "Don't tell your husband." It was true. I felt extremely comfortable there, as if anything good could happen.

We had a sonogram and saw a heartbeat. Since my previous pregnancy we were aware of the complications. We placed a scheduled cerclage at twelve weeks. I went home that day. All was going well.

We still waited to tell the family we were pregnant. I waited this time until four months. We opted for an amniocentesis this time due to our age and wanting to make sure the baby was all right. But I worried about a miscarriage secondary to the amniocentesis. I had the senior OB do the test. I took two days off from work. The amniocentesis went fine. We were just waiting for the results, two weeks. I had no spotting; I still did my bathroom checks JUST in case.

One Saturday I was at a baby shower for a friend. When I got home Jeff said the OB called and said the amniocentesis showed a duplication of the chromosome #6. It usually meant incompatibility with life but they reassured Jeff the pregnancy was going well. I was over twenty weeks; I would have aborted if something were wrong.

The doctors wanted blood-work to check our chromosomes. By this time Jeff was already on the computer, researching chromosomal abnormalities and he found out the baby could have cardiac problems. Multiple sites stated this problem would be incompatible with life.

I went for my blood-work at the OB. Jeff went to two labs because one site only did the test weekly and he didn't want to wait. On July 5th, we had an appointment with a genetic counselor. How ironic, the anniversary of my prior miscarriage.

The genetic counselor discussed our blood chromosomes result. Mine were normal, 46 XX but Jeff has a chromosome inversion on #6, which is the normal same genetic material, just inverted. We laughed when she asked him, "Are you normal?" and he said, "I thought so before this."

The baby's amniocentesis fluid was reevaluated using a solution to stretch the chromosome bands. The test showed a chromosome inversion on # 6 just like Jeff. We found out we were having a boy. We told the family and friends our news. Perfect, a daughter and son.

Jeff kept asking, "Are you OK? Is the baby OK?" I was going to the doctor every two weeks. The baby had a good heartbeat, fetal growth was normal but Jeff and I both felt something was wrong.

The level II sonogram was normal at twenty four weeks. Physically the baby was fine, but neurologically we wouldn't know until he was two. I already knew he would be challenged. I would tell the OB "I feel different, less movement." I was reassured all pregnancies are different, he was breech and the placenta was anterior, making movements different.

Then came September 11, 2001. Devastating news to the world. I just wanted to get home to my family and by four P.M. I was there. As I drove the deserted parkway I thought of all the children who would be without a parent now. At the end of September I went to the OB and my blood pressure was slightly high.

Two weeks later, I went back to the OB, a Friday afternoon; I had a one P.M. appointment. As I was waiting in the examining room I got a sharp pain in my side, so sharp I actually got up and off the table. I thought maybe the baby had moved from the breech position. I told the doctor.

My blood pressure was normal and he was doing the Doppler and couldn't find the heartbeat. I figured the baby had moved in such a way the OB was wasn't picking it up. We went to another exam room.

With the sonogram I knew something was really wrong. There was the baby, still, with no flickering of the heartbeat. I started to cry and must have said a few times, "Are you sure the heart isn't beating?"

A different OB came in for a second opinion and found there was no heartbeat. My fluid was gone; they asked me if I broke my water or was leaking, I said "No." I was so concerned about checking for spotting.

I called Jeff. I remember just wanting to go home. I was so nervous I had to go to the bathroom. While I was in there, I started contracting. Since I had back labor with Elise I had no idea what uterine contractions felt like.

Jeff wanted me to go to the hospital. The doctor took the stitch out, I lost my mucous plug and I starting laboring. The OB was happy it was happening naturally and I didn't have wait. They made all the arrangements at the hospital.

I left the doctor's in disbelief. I called Jeff who would meet me at the hospital, and then my mother. The first question she asked was, "Are you sure?" I said, "I saw the sonogram myself and no heart was beating." She wanted to come to the hospital. I was arguing, "No WE want to be alone. I'll have Jeff call you." Here I was, driving, crying and contracting.

At Winthrop, I was told to go to the New Life Center, the labor and delivery wing. I remember people sitting, waiting for the birth of their grandchild, so happy. Here I was, entering the same area but to deliver a dead baby...MINE.

My OB and a nurse met me. They put their arms around me and said, "I'm sorry." At that moment I felt I would be OK. Their loving touches and soothing voices made me feel safe. As we approached the L&D room I realized this is where I delivered Elise. They said, "We'll go to another room." I said, "No, something good happened here, there's a connection."

I remember sitting on the chair. I called Forever Young (a local baby store) to cancel the delivery of the baby's furniture. I was calm. The nurse wanted to do it, but I needed to. Then Jeff walked in. I could now breakdown. I cried. He kept saying, "It will be OK."

I got into bed and prepared for an epidural. I felt the contractions; the room was quiet, no heart monitors, and just still dim lights. I felt the urge to push. Dr. M. told me it would be slow and to push when I felt the urge. I prayed for little Matthew's spirit to go to someone I knew who was trying to get pregnant. I thought of four women; I didn't want his death to be meaningless. I was grateful for my time of being pregnant with him. Then we talked about the World Trade Center and the anthrax scare. I guess Jeff and the doc spoke. I would just chime in.

I couldn't feel sorry for myself. I needed to care and feel for others and not me.

Then the time approached. I was scared, how was I going to react? How would the baby look? I delivered Matthew with my eyes closed, asking Jeff, "Is everything OK?" The doctor said I did well. I was fine.

He kissed me and told me he would send blood-work to see what happened. He asked if we wanted an autopsy. We said, "Yes, we need some answers."

I delivered Matthew at five sixteen P.M. Jeff and I cried, and then it was my turn to see Matthew and hold him. The nurse brought him in wearing a white gown with blue piping wrapped in a hospital blanket. I held him, his eyes were open, and she tried closing them. He was tiny. He had all his fingers and toes. I just wished he were breathing. Throughout the whole delivery I thought he would be born a miracle and start to cry.

Matthew did look ill, deep down in my heart I guess we always knew. He tried to beat the odds. The nurse asked me if I wanted anything in regard to Matthew. I said his footprints and a lock of his hair. I just wanted him to have everything just like Elise for his memory book. The staff took a few snapshots and professional pictures were taken in his christening dress. Jeff and I both kissed him goodbye. The staff took him away.

I'm crying as I'm typing, it seems like only yesterday. We do miss him.

Jeff called my parents, his dad, his mom and our closest friends, Anthony and Madeline. That's when Jeff actually lost it. The social worker came and spoke to us about burial and gave us literature to read.

The senior doctor told us they might have an answer to Matthew's passing. My blood now showed antibodies to Jka, a rare blood disorder. I didn't have this in my blood in May when I had the cerclage. With Jka, the OB didn't know much but would find someone who did. Jeff and I felt a little better knowing what could have gone wrong. But now we thought, *Could Elise have this?*

I had been here with Elise, a breathing healthy baby and now I had nothing. My son was gone. I remember just wanting to go home but they needed to monitor my blood pressure. Jeff and I cried, hugged, we did little talking. We never slept.

By six A.M. I was officially discharged; they wanted me out before the visiting hours and baby commotion began on the other side. The nurse asked me what I was going to do when I got home. I said, "Jeff will take Elise to her YMCA class." We didn't want her life to be disrupted and wanted it to be normal. Who was I kidding?

We left the hospital with a box, not a baby. It was our memory box with Matthew's Birth and Death Certificate, footprints, snapshot and his christening gown. We left with all the information from the nurse and social worker. At home Shammie, our nanny, and Elise were there. I cried when I saw Shammie; she also had lost a child several years before. With Elise I kept strong.

I found myself reading all the pamphlets the hospital gave me about having a loss. I needed to know others went thorough this.

Jeff was planning Matthew's memorial. I wanted him buried in a park-like setting not a morbid graveyard. Jeff found the perfect place at Pinelawn Cemetery called Babyland. Only children are buried there. The pictures and name sold me; Matthew would be with other kids.

I was scared about the church memorial. I wanted only our immediate family there. I told friends we were keeping it small. There must have been sixty people. I didn't want anyone feeling sorry for me. I started crying as we entered. Elise was twenty two months, holding my hand and telling me it was OK.

I tried sheltering her but she knew her brother died. She carried a tiny doll and basket to church which she never had done before. People hugged me saying, "I'm sorry."

Jeff called me over. Barbara, a friend of my sister-in-law who was trying to get pregnant for ten years, told Jeff in his ear she was pregnant. They both cried. I wished that Matthew's spirit would go to her. Matthew's death had a purpose, a gift to us on his memorial. Father Blood, who married us and baptized Elise, said Mass.

The name we gave Matthew means Gift of God. How I wish he were here. Not a day goes by without us thinking about him.

On October 31, 2001 we went to our first bereavement group. Jeff was reluctant to go. We did Lamaze and birthing classes for Elise, now I needed to do something for Matthew. I felt this was his class. We met a wonderful social worker and friend Anna, and four other couples who grew into family. Jeff said, "I'm doing this for you." In the end we did it for US. Now Jeff was the first to arrive and the last to leave. We shared a lot. I felt guilty being there because I had Elise. The others were first time parents and one couple had multiple losses up to three months.

Anna reassured me, I knew what to expect having Elise and how things would have been for Matthew: a first Christmas, nursing, changing diapers etc. These other parents didn't know. We all grew with each other and shared our intimate life stories no one else would be able to understand. It was a six week session. We added a seventh and then met monthly at one of our homes.

It's been three years and we still see each other. We are there to share the pregnancy stories from trying to conceive, births, baptisms, birthdays and illness. I felt as a family Jeff and I grew stronger and we grew up. We shouldn't be burying a child; it should be the other way around.

Matthew may be gone but he has given us so much. A True Gift of God. I would have preferred him here but God needed him.

On June 11, 2003 we gave birth to our third child, Erica Grace, born four weeks early. She was born blue, eyes opened, cord tightly around her neck but made it through. We thank her Guardian Angel for our miracle.

Erica's Story – Miracles Do Happen

The nearest thing to heaven, you're my angel from above...
so blessed to hold you close.
"Miracle" written by Linda Thompson

After losing Matthew we were referred to an OB specialist at New York University Medical Center who dealt with Jka and antiphospholipid syndrome. On November 27, 2001 we had our appointment. It was Elise's second birthday. Matthew's due date was November 29, 2001.

In the waiting room were tons of photo albums with pictures and heartfelt thank you notes for the miracles since this a high-risk group. The OB's office was a quiet one, the women looked worried and nervous. There was a sigh of relief when they came out of the exam rooms.

Dr. L. took an extensive medical history and reviewed Matthew's autopsy and my blood-work. From Jeff he wanted all his family history. He wanted to do more blood-work to see if things changed since Matthew's delivery.

The nurse in the lab asked me if I'd eaten. I said, "Just coffee this morning," thinking they wanted a fasting blood-work. Then she comes back with peanut butter crackers and juice and says, "We need a lot of blood, so start eating. I don't want you passing out."

Jeff looked at all the tubes to be filled, a rainbow of colors. He asked, "Are all those blood tubes for me or the both of us?" They drew about fifteen to twenty tubes from me.

We ask when we can we start trying to get pregnant. He advised six months, so we could grieve, perhaps longer. I remember saying to myself *I'm fine, I'm handling this well, we can start trying; another pregnancy will make me feel better*. In reality, Jeff and I were sacred to death.

Our support group was ending the week of Christmas. We were strong while attending group and then like Anna said, it's a roller coaster of feelings, low and high.

I remember when group first started; we were going to put up a tree for Elise. We didn't want her to suffer. We didn't have the desire to or the strength, but she was too young to understand. We needed to remember Matthew and the true meaning of the holiday, not the commercial part.

The doctors confirmed their suspicions; it was a clotting disorder: Antiphospholipid syndrome and Jka antibodies to the fetus. With the next pregnancy they would start anti-coagulation therapy and monitor the fetus for hydrops for the Jka.

We survived the holidays. The support group ended, but we all kept in touch. For the first few months we met monthly for coffee or dinner. There were phone calls or emails. I remember Rosemary was in a SPALS group. That was my goal: to become pregnant and to join the next group.

It was like getting promoted. We were trying to conceive but then we chickened out. I couldn't bear to lose another child. In January I joined Weight Watchers, I was tired of having this pregnancy weight or baby fat without a baby. I wanted to get healthy before getting pregnant.

By May my morale was up, I lost a lot of weight. I felt good about me. We took family trips in April, May, June and August. Maybe we were trying not to feel the pain that Matthew would have been five months for our trip to Florida. I kept doing these mind games: if he was here this is how it would be.

By the summer we wanted another child.

I saw my OB in June. Each time I saw him, three months later I was pregnant. I went for a check-up and everything was OK, see you in six months. I knew when I was ovulating and nothing was happening.

In October a friend said, "Let's go to St. Gerard's church in Port Jefferson Station." She went there as a child. The first Sunday of the month they give a special blessing for all couples trying to conceive and who are pregnant. Diane and I went to the fountain, just the two of us. I became emotional when the priest said, "For all the children who have gone." I thought of Matthew. We received a candle and a prayer card with a green ribbon and St. Gerard medal for those trying to conceive. As we were leaving the church the priest congratulated me. I told Diane I had the green ribbon, not the red meaning I conceived.

On October 12th we had Matthew's anniversary mass on his first birthday in heaven. We sent balloons up and remembered. At the end of October we attended Winthrop University Hospital's first pregnancy loss conference and memorial service.

We met our old friends from group there and new couples. It was nice seeing all who had gone on to have healthy pregnancies and deliveries. The guest speaker spoke about antiphospholipid syndrome. I remember Jeff asking tons of questions. I remember feeling doomed we wouldn't have another baby. The speakers spoke about retrieving the eggs, fertilizing them and keeping the healthy ones. Jeff said, "That's what we will do."

A week went by, no period. I did a pregnancy test thinking *I'm stressed we aren't pregnant, I feel no different.* Well it was POSITIVE!

I didn't want anyone knowing. I kept thinking, *What if it's a blighted ovum or it's a false positive*? I didn't do any blood-work on myself; I was a true patient. We met with Dr. R. He reviewed my chart, and then suggested a sonogram. There was the flickering of the heartbeat. Jeff and I cried.

We were about eight weeks along. I was calmer after seeing the heartbeat. It was my thirty-sixth birthday and I felt this was the best gift ever.

I continued with the prenatal vitamins and started a baby aspirin regimen for the clotting disorder. I was given a prescription to start Fragmin, a low molecular Heparin, to prevent my blood from getting too thick and to prevent formation of a blood clot. Jeff and I were happy but petrified. We couldn't bear losing another baby but we knew it could happen.

I started spotting the day of the first SPALS meeting. I told Monica, the social worker, this might be my last meeting because I felt I was going to have a miscarriage. Patty and Jenny reassured me this happened to them in the beginning and now they were each in the sixteenth week and doing well.

Jeff never wanted to go to the prenatal loss meetings when we lost Matthew. This time he asked me, "When are we going to the SPALS meeting?"

It was our venting time; we were with people with the same fears and hopes of having a living child. Jeff was the only guy in the beginning.

He would tell me, "I'm not going. I feel stupid," but deep down he wanted to go. So at one of the meetings I mentioned it to the group and Patty joked with him about being the only man. As months passed a member's husband who never came to prenatal loss groups came to SPALS. It was at times a joking, laughing group and sometimes the stress level and fears were so high you could feel the tension. When a member would deliver it was a sigh of relief; another baby made it!

I told the OB I was a nervous wreck. I was spotting. He did a sonogram and the heart was beating. I always had to first know the baby was OK then we could proceed. The OB said something comforting to me, "You will always worry first while you are pregnant, after your delivery, when they're little, in grammar school, high school…." How right he was!

I was doing the Fragmin injections daily; the doctor was checking my blood level monthly to see if the amount of Fragmin was sufficient for preventing a clot. The test is called an anti factor X.

We had an amniocentesis done at sixteen weeks and the fluid was sent to a lab to see if the baby had Jka antibodies.

In two weeks we found out we were having a girl and she had the Jka antibodies. We were happy we were having a girl since Elise, our first, was a girl and she made it.

A part of us wanted a boy; not to replace Matthew, but in a way to memorialize him. We both thought before we found out the gender, *If it were a boy, would we lose him, too*? Is something with my body rejecting a boy, or would I always compare, *This is what Matthew would have been like*?

Our SPALS group met biweekly and kept us focused.

At the next OB appointment I met another doctor in the practice for the first time. I explained my story as he was reviewing my paperwork. He had his back towards me and was focusing on the chart. He kept shaking his head in disbelief. Jeff and I looked at each other and thought, *What's with this guy*? He made us feel as if we were doomed. Jeff said, "Doc, it's a complicated case." The doctor looked at his fingernails and shaking his head said, "You're not kidding."

I chimed in, "Am I one of your worst patients?" He said, "Yes." This is a Harvard graduate with no bedside manner; he seemed like the Mad Scientist. "Let's check to see if your cervix is shortening." He did an internal sonogram and the length of my cervix was fine. This time they wanted to evaluate the cervical length and not place a cerclage.

I said, "Doc, that's good." He replied, "For now."

We left the exam room. I saw one of the nurses and said, "What's with him?" She said, "I know he's the 'salt of the earth'," (a nickname for him). He was thorough and knew a lot about Jka and antiphospholipid syndrome.

With these problems, we were at NYU every other week. Over an hour drive each way. We continued with a sonogram every two weeks, anti factor X blood-work monthly, cervical checks every two weeks until twenty eight weeks. It was at this point that the doctors felt if the baby came it had a good chance of survival.

At thirty weeks the fun started. We went to NYU weekly for non-stress tests (NST, usually a monitoring of the baby's movements), MCA (middle cerebral artery) Doppler and fetal growth level. At the non-stress test station, Olga, the nurse, asked me, "Have you felt the baby move?" I said, "At times but rarely." With an anterior placenta and history of fetal loss the only thing I wished was to have this baby move. She handed me the clicker and she said, "When you feel the baby move click the button." I could hear the baby's heart beat, which was reassuring to me. Depending on how I was sitting the heartbeat was getting louder, lower, or I would simply lose the sound. Finally after forty five minutes the tracing was fine. I was reassured, until the following week.

Thank goodness for SPALS. Over the course of my pregnancy, many of the members had delivered and that was reassuring.

One Sunday morning at St. Gerard's, I was in the bathroom, when a woman said, "Congratulations! Is this your first?" I said, "No it's my third. I have a daughter and lost my son." I began to cry and told her why I was coming to Mass here the first Sunday of the month. She comforted me, saying she would add my name to the prayer list.

I don't know why I opened up to this woman. Usually I would say it's my second pregnancy and not mention Matthew, but that day I was thirty three weeks pregnant with Erica and I was thinking of Matthew. This was the week of pregnancy when I lost him. I went up for the blessing and I remember feeling the baby move. I was grateful since I wasn't feeling anything prior to this moment. Then I thought, *What if the baby moved and the cord was around her neck, this could be a sign something bad was happening.*

Being pregnant and getting to the week when I lost Matthew was EXTREMELY scary.

I remember telling the doctor we would rather have this baby out than in. We discussed having an amniocentesis at thirty seven weeks. If the lungs were developed the induction would be the next day.

Now reality was setting in. I was in denial for the whole pregnancy, going back and forth to doctors. I felt more as if we were treating an ailment. I wished I could have been one of those pregnant women who are happy, naive, and in the pregnancy bliss, instead of being a worrywart.

Thursday of the thirty-seventh week we scheduled the amniocentesis and Friday we would deliver with the doctor who had been shaking his head in disbelief, "old salt of the earth." We now felt comfortable with him and had become friends as he turned out to be a caring, honest, knowledgeable, bright individual.

I was nervous about having an amniocentesis so late in the pregnancy, thinking, *What if they puncture the baby's heart?* I worried, but many women had amniocentesis for lung maturity and they do well with the procedure.

I went for a non-stress test and the MCA. The tech did the scan and plotted the values. She discussed the results with the radiologist. The Chief of Radiology came in and said the scans were abnormal; the baby was in the gray zone. He would call the OB and advised getting the baby out now. There should be an amniocentesis today not later in the week.

Jeff and I spoke to the OB who said, "Let's do the amniocentesis now. We will have the results by two A.M. and will deliver the baby."

I had all these "what if" questions: What if the lungs aren't developed, what do we do? What does this gray zone mean? What if I am forming a clot?

He kept reassuring me, "Let's do the amniocentesis first. I'll call with the results and then we will take the next step."

As I was being scanned he had a hard time finding a pouch to insert the needle. Picture this: on the right side on my stomach, closer to the breast, it was high up by a rib. I was scared. He kept telling me to relax. I was watching the monitor.

I closed my eyes when the needle went in, he got the fluid. But there was some bleeding in the pouch so they scanned me for thirty minutes to make sure the baby wasn't in any distress and repeated the non-stress test.

We left NYU in early evening with Elise asleep in the car. I remember Jeff and I were worried. Should I have asked to be admitted? Jeff was trying to make light of the situation. "Let's get a bite to eat," he said which meant he had an appetite. Jeff said, "By tomorrow night, the baby will be here."

That night, who slept? A friend of mine gave me a St. Gerard cloth to put on my belly when praying. It was tucked in my nightstand drawer for the delivery. I got it out, put it on my belly, and prayed. I prayed to Matthew to keep his sister safe.

At eight thirty A.M. the nurse called, "The lungs are mature, come on in, you're having your baby today." We couldn't believe it; the time had come. I finally packed my bag that morning after getting the news.

In the labor room I was put on the fetal monitor. We heard the baby's heartbeat, music to my ears.

The anesthesiologist placed the epidural catheter in my back, the OB broke my water, and Pitocin to contract my uterus was started. At twelve thirty P.M. the nurse evaluated me and I was crowning, the baby's head was down. The OB came and the room was being transformed to a delivery suite with monitors.

I started to push, it seemed forever. I was tired from the past two days and now I needed to push this child out. I heard the OB say, "Get the vacuum!" The baby was having a lot of decelerations. Jeff told me, "Nancy, the head is out! Just one more push," and the doctor agreed with him. One more push.

She came out not crying, blue-tinged. I'm asking Jeff, "Is she OK?" He didn't answer. Finally the doctor cut part of the cord that was tightly wound around her neck. She began to cry, and so did I. She's here and alive! Then Jeff cut the cord. The Pediatric resident checked the baby. He put the baby in my arms, it was a miracle!

Erica Grace! Miracles do happen.

Our Winthrop family was called; Anna sent a beautiful email announcement. It felt as if we graduated. I remember always reading the emails and thinking *I can't wait to belong to the SPALS group*. Thanks to Anna, Margaret and Monica for their support and time. I dedicate my stories to our babies, the ones we lost and for the ones to come.

AMY

Solomon's Flowers

I'm standing on foundation and have no farther to fall.
Smilla's Sense of Snow written by Peter Hoeg

From my kitchen window I can just about see the green shoots on Solomon's flowers. I call them Solomon's flowers because I planted them after I lost the second baby, early October 2000. Solomon's flowers are fighters, just like Solomon was. They pushed through the hard earth when the temperature here was in the mid-thirties. I don't even remember what I planted, tulips maybe. It's just as well. I can barely remember how I survived my nightmare.

My journey started on March 5, 2000, a typical Sunday night. I was in bed watching TV with Eric. The new game show "Who Wants to be a Millionaire" was all the rage and I was pretty good at it. I knew if I just could somehow become a contestant on the show, an easy $32,000 could be won without my even using a lifeline. I would buy our baby the most wonderful things and take a long maternity leave from my job. I was hungry, being almost five months pregnant and all. And I did something I never do: I ate in bed. A big no-no in my book, for my dad drummed into my head for years, "No eating in your room." Not only was I eating in my bedroom, I was sitting in my bed, tucked in under the down comforter, munching on a bowl of Cheerios.

I must have fallen asleep after the game show ended. I remember Eric channel-surfing and seeing bits of various programs, a mini-series on the 1980s, some racing cars, the weather. I remember dreaming about water and feeling wet. And then I woke up.

I was wet. Everything around me was wet. My underwear, my pajamas, the sheet — everything. I thought I was bleeding. I'd had spotting all through the almost twenty weeks of pregnancy and even had one episode of a minor placental abruption. I wasn't supposed to worry about losing our baby but somehow I knew I was in trouble. I flew down the stairs of our home to the only bathroom we had. While running I was leaking big time. I could feel it rushing down my legs and couldn't get to the bathroom fast enough. I sat on the toilet and heard a plop. I was terrified to look but when I did, I didn't see red or a baby as I'd thought I would. I saw some gray fluid and tissue. I wanted to be relieved.

I went back upstairs to the bedroom and told Eric something was wrong. I phoned the medical service who paged my doctor. I told him I thought I'd passed my mucous plug because that was the only thing I could think could have happened. I didn't read far enough in the *What to Expect While You Are Expecting* to know exactly what happens when you pass your mucous plug. My doctor sent me to the emergency room of the hospital.

Sitting shocked in the ER waiting room I was amazed at how helpless I was. I wasn't a candidate to go to the labor and delivery ward, as I wasn't yet twenty weeks pregnant. Such an arbitrary determination! To this day I still wonder if some other outcome could have been achieved if I'd just been sent to L&D.

After waiting for what seemed like hours I finally was taken back into the ER to have a sonogram. The resident had me undress so he could do an internal exam as well. Up on the screen, there was our baby, alive and kicking and pounding away, as I'd seen so many times previously. He or she was such an active little thing. *Hurray!* I thought. But right there on the resident's face was 'the look.' He must have known right then. I wouldn't have this baby.

My OB arrived and I was admitted. After I was settled in, Eric went home to get some sleep, feed our three cats and gear up for the day ahead.

When I woke in the morning, I discovered my roommate had just given birth to twins. *How ironic* I thought as here I was, desperately trying just to have one baby. I'm sure I fantasized about her giving me one of her babies. I had another sonogram in the afternoon and my baby was still alive, but I had lost most of my amniotic fluid. Unless it was restored in my uterus, our baby would die. My options were discussed.

What hell. I'd had a full preterm premature rupture of membranes (pprom), something most women have after thirty seven weeks. At this point there is very little done to save the pregnancy and most doctors will work to save the mother. I remember crying for hours.

This was Monday. My mother came to see me, my dad and my grandma came, friends of my parents, and my friend Terry. I called my boss and some of my friends. I needed prayers, for me, for the baby, for everything. I felt I was losing not only the baby, but my mind as well.

I think the prostaglandin suppositories to begin my labor were started Monday evening. They were to be given every few hours until my cervix dilated to five centimeters and I could deliver. This wasn't what I'd planned. This was supposed to be a wonderful experience, having my first child. Instead, I was in the hospital, crying, with my Dad sleeping in the bed beside me so Eric could get some rest at home.

I was given some reading material about pregnancy loss on Tuesday, as I was still not dilated. I requested to see a Rabbi and would have settled for any member of the clergy. Rabbi P. walked in. An Orthodox Rabbi, a short man with a black hat and payis, who sat in a chair across the room from me while I cried and asked questions about why this was happening to me. The Rabbi explained God had a soul whom he needed to place for a short period of time, and he chose me. I thought this made sense and clung to it, as if I was doing something noble.

I felt our baby kick for the last time around five P.M. on Tuesday. I decided I wouldn't stroke my stomach anymore or try to get our baby to move. I had to stop paying attention to the life inside of me. I had to move beyond thinking and being a pregnant woman. I started to pray I would dilate already and get this ordeal over with. Little did I know, this was just the beginning.

Wednesday morning, March 8, the contractions started. They hurt a lot. And to think I didn't even have to dilate to ten centimeters as if I was at full term. I took a shot of Demerol and that hurt. But at least I could get some rest.

My friend's aunt called to comfort me. She said, "Do you know what a vitamin does? It gives you strength. I will be your vitamin today."

Near three P.M. my OB told me I was just about ready to start pushing. *Was he crazy?* If I pushed and delivered this baby then I wouldn't be pregnant anymore and I wouldn't be a mommy and there wouldn't be anything special about me. How could my doctor ask me to do that?

But with Eric behind me holding onto my arms and my back, and my OB in front of me, in just a few pushes, I delivered my baby. My whole world collapsed. I remember hearing the silence in the room, and then the sobs of some woman crying and it took a minute to realize that woman was me. I remember how sad my OB looked and how thankful I was I didn't have to see Eric's face. I clung to Eric's arm as if I was going to float off into the universe. I'd never failed so much before in all my life.

Our baby was taken away since I had instructed the staff I didn't want to see it, nor did I want to know what it was. This was the advice given by the floor nurses. Looking back I wonder if the L&D nurses would have advised otherwise.

I immediately asked for a social worker consult and to be allowed to get up and go to the bathroom. I wanted out of the hospital so badly. I'd been in the hospital room, in the hospital bed for over three days straight. I'd eaten nothing except green Jell-O, once, in three days. I put on the raggedy old sweatpants Eric brought for me. I refused to be escorted to the hospital exit in a wheelchair. *Why bother?* This wasn't the joyous 'new mom leaving the hospital with baby in arms Kodak moment' it was supposed to be. I was suffocating and just needed to be outside.

Walking through the hospital doors I was struck by the streetlights in the darkness. I had no sense four hours had passed since my delivery. I just wanted to be at home. Eric opened the sofa-bed in the living room for me since I wasn't allowed to climb the stairs for a few days. I remember answering the telephone and cursing out a telemarketer. Didn't he know I'd just given birth to a dead baby? What the fuck was wrong with the world? How could he ask me to think about changing my long-distance carrier on a night like this?

I lay at home for days crying and feeling sorry for myself. In the extra ten days I took off from work, I had to figure out how to go on with my life. Nothing really mattered to me. I was post-partum, bleeding, hormonal and grieving. My breast milk came in. Wasn't that a trip? I got to sit around with icepacks on my breasts to make the milk go away. It was probably then I learned not to ask, "What else could go wrong?" since it seemed something else always could.

I came home on a Wednesday and Alex, my stepson, was coming to stay for the weekend. He wasn't even five years old. He couldn't wait to be a big brother. Now what was I supposed to do? As things evolved I was the one who told him the baby had died and wouldn't be coming to live with us. He looked so sad and so serious and wanted reassurance I was OK. Alex would turn out to be a true friend to me on this journey.

I thought I could be like Eric, just walk out of the hospital and not look back, focus on healing and getting pregnant again. What a joke. That was definitely not my M.O. I angrily called the Social Work office at the hospital as I'd been told I could do. I was thankful no one was there to answer my call; the anonymity of the answering machine was wonderful. Within a few days, Anna called me back. I remember feeling very hostile and bitchy on the telephone. She told me she had a support group forming for other women in my position. *My position*? I thought. What was that? A failure at womanhood? Cows, dogs, even cockroaches manage to have children and here I'd lost the most precious thing to me in the world. I was nothing. I told Anna I would try to come but I wasn't going to stay in a room with other women just crying for an hour.

There were four couples in the group. And as we went around sharing out stories we all were trying to be brave. We all were sad. We all were grieving. One couple had two miscarriages after a successful pregnancy. Another lost a full-term girl. And the last couple had struggled through years of infertility, and then lost twin girls, in the same manner I lost my baby. In the first group session you could see the walls coming down, just a little.

The group came to be my lifeline. For its six week duration, we touched on so many issues, our physical and emotional health, how we felt about our bodies, other people's support or lack thereof. We were all at different places on our journeys. I hadn't even been given the green light to start trying to get pregnant again. And then I had to miss one of the sessions, and that mentally set me back.

My physical nightmare hadn't ended. At seven weeks post-partum, I had one period that wouldn't stop. As I was losing blood clots the size of my fist, my doctor sent me to the ER of a different hospital, thank goodness. And because of the bleeding, I had to have a D&C, as apparently there were still 'products of conception' in my uterus. And all I was thinking as I was lying on the gurney in the ER is, *Why me, why again? What is wrong with me?* Eric, loving as he could, tried to lift my spirits. We shared a joke between us and I almost believed things would turn out all right.

The morning after the D&C, I spoke to Anna. Amazingly, I was physically feeling much better. I told her I needed her help. I decided I wanted to know who the baby was and if there was anything I could have from the hospital. I needed her to get it for me.

A few days later, back at work, I called her and she told me something wonderful. I'd had a baby boy. I suspected all along the baby was a boy and I'd been right. I actually cried tears of joy at my desk. I named him Solomon, which means peace. He was six and a half inches long and weighed about thirteen ounces. I just couldn't give him the boy name Eric and I'd picked out because I still harbored some hope I would have a son someday.

At the next support group, Anna gave me a Certificate of Birth, not a legal Birth Certificate, but something I could complete and keep. She also gave me a baby blanket in a memory box. Many times I cuddled with the blanket for comfort, even though I knew it wasn't Solomon's blanket. And the best gift of all I received: pictures of Solomon after his birth. He was perfectly formed from what I could tell. His skin was very dark and his eyes were still fused shut. He would have been born with a full head of hair. He looked surprisingly like my brother Michael. And I just fell in love.

My depression continued, more severely now since I'd seen my son and knew what I'd lost. One Sunday morning Eric left the house to play softball. Alex was watching TV downstairs. Lying in bed, I stared at the painkillers (from the D&C) on my dresser and tried to calculate how many footsteps I needed to take to get to them, how many I would have to take to join Solomon, how quick my journey would be. I didn't want to die but I couldn't think of another way to be with my baby. I snapped out of my fantasy as Alex yelled for me to come downstairs.

By the time group ended, it was Mother's Day. And although many determined I wasn't a mother by their definition, I made the decision I was. Even though my child hadn't lived, I still had given birth. I had had dreams for my child from the second I knew he existed. I just felt like a mom. Eric gave me a gold little boy charm and it never left my neck for the next seventeen months.

June arrived and it was time for Barb's baby shower. Barb is my best friend. We've known each other since high school. We attended college together. We both married for love the first time around and even for love the second time around. She was pregnant, due three days after I was due with Solomon. I didn't know what to do. The pain of going to the shower would pierce through me like a knife. And the pain of letting down Eric and Barb and her husband Jon if I didn't go was even worse. So I went. And it was as horrible and as wonderful as I expected.

Barb was absolutely beautiful. I quickly surmised what I would look like if it were me. Her aunt kindly put me to work helping out in the kitchen. Before the party started, Barb and I had a few minutes alone. We talked about Solomon and my loss and I shared my pictures and we shared our tears. At times during the party I just had to excuse myself, the pain was too much. I cried in her bathroom more than once and then composed myself to rejoin the party. But I knew I'd made the right decision, for my friend and for myself.

As July approached, I became more and more depressed. Eric, Alex and I were invited to a friend's house for a July 4th celebration. These were good friends but I'd taken so much already, from them and from others, I declined attending and insisted Eric and Alex go.

My friend just couldn't understand what I meant when I told her, "Eric wouldn't be able to support me enough to get through this." She took this to mean Eric was being unsupportive but what I meant was, "I'm not strong enough to deal with all the stupid and careless remarks coming my way, albeit unintentional, but still hurtful just the same; I want Eric to relax and have a good time."

July 28th was my due date. A few days before, Eric and I traveled to Washington, D.C. I didn't want to be at home. On that morning, in the hotel room, I fantasized someone would knock on the door and hand me a baby. It didn't materialize and I cried deep sobs, like after Solomon's delivery. Eric held me and let me cry.

Four months after my loss another dipstick said I was pregnant. Wow, what luck! So while I grieved the loss of Solomon, I tried to keep sane about this new pregnancy. I found an online web-ring for women pregnant after loss (SPALS) and joined immediately. The camaraderie was comforting. I wasn't alone. There were almost four hundred women on the list. Some were waiting to try again to get pregnant, some were trying to get pregnant and some were trying to get through an agonizing pregnancy. I'd found another tool to help me with my grief.

Sad to say, I lost this baby to a blighted ovum. Baby Z as I referred to it, didn't really take. A sonogram revealed only an empty gestational sac, no baby. I started to wonder what I'd done to deserve all this. I broke down in the prep room at the hospital, waiting for my next D&C. After providing the nurse with my 'loss history 101,' she did the most incredible thing. She walked over to my side and just held my hand. The comfort and warmth of another human right then alleviated so much of my heartache.

I was back to the drawing board. I couldn't really grieve for this baby whom I learned would have also been a boy. I was numb and beaten down. I was supposed to wait another two months before trying to conceive again.

Even though group had ended, I continued to see Anna about once a month. She was happy I was pregnant again, and saddened I'd experienced another loss. I confessed to having numerous arguments with Eric and about wanting to just give up. I knew I was living my life in some sort of haze. There were weeks I felt I had no control in my life. Anna tried to jumpstart my mind and suggested planting some flowers. I normally don't do the outdoors; I'm not a nature lover. I don't like bugs or dirt. But I needed to find something to do, to renew life, to find a new normal, and luckily there was still some time left in New York for the fall planting season. So off to the Garden Center I went.

I perused the bulbs and gardening tools. I picked some red, some orange and some purple flowers. These were the colors I thought I'd like to see. I picked two trees in our backyard and a strip of grass alongside our driveway, and on a pleasant early November afternoon, I started digging. Pulling out the dirt hurt my hands but dropping in the bulbs made me feel productive in some way. I wouldn't have my babies but I'd always be able to think about them when I see the flowers bloom each spring.

Hark, Alison Is Born

Not everyone understands how you can spin two lassos at the same time,
one of hope and one of grief.
Vanishing Acts written by Jodi Picoult

On August 14, 2001 I was reborn. I felt at peace with my husband, my family, my friends, the world and myself. This was the day Alison was born.

It seems as if Alison had been waiting to be born forever. I'd endured the loss of my son, Solomon, and another baby, who would have been a boy, too. There I was in the operating room of Plainview Hospital when I had a transformation. I'd heard childbirth can change your life, but for me it wasn't in the way it is for most other women.

I wasn't supposed to get pregnant yet. But after two losses in five months, the thought of waiting another thirty days…well my OB might as well have told me to wait thirty years. Waiting seemed an impossible task. Toni Weschlers's book *Taking Charge of Your Fertility* became my bible. I read it every day. I charted my temperature every morning at five thirty A.M. To this day, whenever I take my temperature, I can't hear the 'beep beep' when the temperature is completed without feeling compelled to write it down on a chart. Finally I knew I was ovulating. This was the second time after I lost the second one. I was obsessed with having a baby.

After "baby-dancing" with Eric, I lay on the couch, trying to position my hips appropriately to increase my chances of conception. This is what women obsessed with becoming pregnant do. We use charts, ovulation predictors, cough medicine, pelvic positioning and all kinds of other tactics to achieve our goals. We wish each other fertile vibes and baby dust. We sit on chairs pregnant women have just sat on. And I was no different. My goal in life was to have a baby.

I was still charting my temperature after day twenty eight of my cycle. Some online computer software I was using kept telling me I was probably not pregnant. My good old hand-written chart had another story to tell. And then there were the omens.

I don't know if I was always superstitious but I became so after I lost Solomon. I tried to read clues to my life into everything. One of my first inklings I might be pregnant was an empty shoebox. Eric thought I was ridiculous when I told him this. I'd kept the mementos of my previous pregnancies in shoeboxes: doctor's appointment cards, sonogram pictures, test results, sympathy cards. I'd just bought boots and there was this box lying around, just waiting. It seemed like an omen to me that I had a shoebox available.

The next sign occurred during Christmas week in Florida at my mother-in-law's house, I saw some gray hairs on my head. I don't mean one here and another there. But on the right side of my head as I was pulling the hairbrush through my hair, there were tons! The only other times I noticed these assemblies of gray hairs was when I'd been pregnant. I really started to think I was pregnant and Eric really started to consider institutionalizing me.

And then I had an intense urge to throw up. I made a mad dash to the bathroom. And there wasn't a thing. Nothing but a metallic taste in my mouth. I pretty much knew then.

We arrived home from Florida on New Year's Eve. Was I ever so glad to get this year over. In a nutshell, it had sucked. I'd endured so much physically and mentally. I just needed some peace.

New Year's Day 2001. Two lines on the stick meant I was pregnant. I was thrilled! I ran to kiss Eric and tell him the good news. He was thrilled as always and I secretly hoped he was starting to understand what I was doing with my charting and my shoebox and my hair. I called Barb and her husband Jon to tell them the good news because 1) I figured they would be happy for us and 2) they would help us through our grief when we lost this baby.

Another journey had begun. I was still confused and was still grieving. I didn't have the answers as to why I'd lost Solomon or Baby Z. I'd had all kinds of tests and group counseling and individual counseling for months. I'd been beaten down, risen up, only to be beaten down yet again. And here I was, not only at the amusement park for another trip but on the freaking carousel for the third time. Grief is often referred to as a roller coaster; it has its ups and downs. I see it as a merry-go-round: not only do you endure the ups and downs, you are going around and around at the same time. It was very disorienting.

I made up my mind this pregnancy would have to be different. As it was, I was no longer employed. Alex needed some changes in his life and I was the fallback gal. I was able to spend my entire pregnancy at home, relaxing with my feet up, popping bonbons. If only that were the case.

The mental anguish I went through for the whole nine months and the physical sickness I went through for the first five made me wonder if I was out of my mind. People had told me if they'd gone through the first loss, they would have never tried again to get pregnant. That just wasn't me. I had to have a baby. It became THE singular purpose of my life. If I could have had a baby by sheer determination, I would have. But it doesn't work that way.

I would spend the next several months living two existences: the first of a woman grieving the loss of a baby and anxious as all hell, and the second as a pregnant woman. Most of the time, I was the former but to the outside world, I was the latter. I spent my entire pregnancy checking the toilet paper after going to the bathroom, convinced at any time I would find blood and my dream would be over yet again. I was pregnant for nine months, which is roughly 270 days. I went to the bathroom on average seven times a day, almost 1900 wipe-checks. I'm convinced this isn't something normal pregnant women go through. I spent nine months terrified. And I know the morning sickness I endured was exacerbated by my mental state, but I couldn't help it.

It was suspected I lost Solomon due to an incompetent cervix so my OB decided to put in a cerclage to hold my cervix closed. To be truthful I would have done just about anything to have this baby and had often told people if I needed to stand on my head for the whole nine months I would.

March 2nd I was lying in the triage room hysterical, and I didn't know if the grief had gotten hold of me, or the reality that this might possibly work, and in five months I might have a child. Eric was great, running interference for me with the staff who I knew thought I'd lost my mind. The phlebotomy technician believed she'd caused me great pain inserting my IV because I couldn't stop crying. There was also a woman behind curtain number two in labor and I could hear the fetal monitor and the baby's heartbeat and I wanted so badly for it to be me. And when the midwife came to listen to my baby's heartbeat, she couldn't find it. The tears kept flowing; from the grief, from the discomfort of the IV and additionally from the mauling of my stomach as all the nurses and techs tried desperately to find the baby's heartbeat. They reminded me I was only fourteen weeks pregnant and this was very common.

I walked into the OR, which was such a different experience than delivering a stillborn in a hospital room. As the nurses started prepping me I reminded them I must hear the baby's heartbeat before they did anything. I was trying to be rational and reasonable, not paranoid. My thinking was, *Why go through this if the baby has died or some how escaped*? I was lying down and looking at the oversized operating room clock and after five excruciatingly long minutes, the nurse-midwife found it. Hurray! A huge sigh of relief. Now for my spinal. One needle into my spine was all it took and I numbed from the waist down. A surreal experience as I watched my OB and another doctor move my legs up and down and to the sides. I felt nothing. It was very freaky.

While waiting in Recovery for the feeling to return to my body, I ask to see the baby. I needed to make sure the spinal, the surgery and my hysteria hadn't hurt it or worse. The nurse wheeled in the portable sonogram machine and there the baby was, alive and kicking. I scarfed down the fish and spinach lunch the hospital provided and Eric took me home.

Upon getting home from the cerclage surgery, I barely made it to the bathroom. I lost my lunch so violently I couldn't even clean it up. I went to bed and couldn't even deal with the television or the radio being on. My parents came over for dinner to offer moral support, to check on me, and to bring me chocolates. I wasn't supposed to indulge in them but I did. And then the guilt I felt convinced me I had lost the baby and I cried. Too much caffeine is a no-no and I knew this. Not only had I put the baby in danger, I did so knowingly, which convinced me I would lose the baby.

The cerclage surgery was on Friday. By Sunday afternoon I had a headache. And it wasn't one of those "take two aspirins and call me in the morning" headaches. It was a "have you ever had an anvil dropped on your head?" headache. It was a spinal headache. Apparently there is a one in a gazillion chance I could have this problem with the spinal anesthesia and that's me, the poster child for one in a gazillion. So I couldn't move my head off the pillow or stand up for more than a minute. After speaking with my OB and the anesthesiologist, I decided I could tolerate some Tylenol and a little bit of cola in lieu of a stronger prescription painkiller. Apparently the caffeine from the box of chocolates did nothing at all to stem this but some caffeine from soda might help. Sure enough it slowly worked and once the pain was completely gone, after about ten days, I went back to being merely paranoid about losing this baby.

A few days after my cerclage was the anniversary of Solomon. The headache and nausea compounded my heartache and I couldn't bear to get out of bed. I looked through the memory box of sonogram pictures and sympathy cards. I think I had handled everything very well. Then I came across a book Alex made in daycare about his family. He'd drawn several pages explaining his life at his mom's and his life with Eric and me. The second to last page was just about me. Alex had drawn me at the baby hospital where I was having a sonogram. This set off a crying jag so severe I was sure the baby wouldn't survive. When I pulled myself together, I found a little peace writing a letter to Solomon in my journal. I poured out my grief and told Solomon about all the things going on in our lives. I hoped he was watching over me.

By May, I looked pregnant, and slowly was making the transition from XL clothes for normal people to maternity clothes. And there is something that happens to women when they are pregnant, maybe it's by default, but maternity clothes start to look attractive. The times I wasn't pregnant I thought they were pretty darn ugly. So I bought some clothes in the appropriate maternity size and tried to convince myself I'd actually get to wear them. I'd just about stretched out every pair of leggings and sweatpants I'd owned. I was bursting out of Eric's XL shirts that I wore longer than I should have because I was convinced if I did anything different, like wear maternity clothes, I would lose the baby.

Family and friends were starting to pester me about registering. And I was thinking, *Why on earth would I do that? I may have this big belly and five sonogram pictures but did they honestly think I was having a baby, with my track record and all?*

And another friend scolded me for not wearing something red every-day, a bendel.

On Mother's Day, Eric and I went to a Judaica store and purchased a bendel from Jerusalem. In the car, Eric attached the bendel to my wrist. Then we went to Babies R Us and began our registry. It was enlightening and for this one afternoon, the first time ever during the pregnancy, I allowed myself to feel and act as a normal pregnant woman. I walked around with the electronic scanner, scanning barcodes all over the store. I even dared to put baby clothing on my registry even though the store clerks said not to. I had to be bold, was my thinking. This may be all that comes of this pregnancy and I was desperate to find a little pleasure.

As we left Babies R Us, I realized the bendel was gone, lost somewhere in the store. I cried in the car the entire twenty-minute ride home. I immedi-ately pulled out my sewing box and attached a red thread to my ankle. I was frantic I'd jinxed the baby.

At this point, I was feeling a new anxiety as I passed my loss-point (nineteen weeks and six days) when I lost Solomon. I was convinced almost every second I would lose the baby. I was scared to go out, to drive, to just be normal, whatever that was. I spent a lot of time on the Internet, on a closed email list for women who are pregnant after loss.

The online SPALS group became my best friend, as these women knew what I was going through and were going through the same things them-selves. Here I could live the dual personality I'd cultivated for months and these women didn't think I was nuts. As much as Eric and Barb and my mom and my brother tried to understand, I know they meant well but there were organic limitations to their understanding. I didn't feel safe unloading my worries with them. They might break under the weight of my fears.

I became obsessed with feeling the baby move. I lay down constantly on my left side. In fact, I spent the greater part of the day lying down on my left side. If I didn't feel the baby move when I wanted it to move I panicked. Then I drank some orange juice and talked to my stomach and tried to coax the baby into moving. Earlier on in the pregnancy, the staff at my OB's office convinced me not to buy a baby Doppler to listen to the baby's heartbeat. I knew they were right, as I would have been in their office constantly because of what would have been my inability to find the baby's heartbeat. And only once during the nine months did I make an urgent call to my OB's office and insist I had to come in to hear the baby's heartbeat. The invitation stood for me to come in anytime, as the staff knew I was frightened.

By now I had had seven or eight sonograms, all of which showed a normally growing baby inside a normal looking uterus. I accumulated twenty nine pictures. The baby had all its parts. One technician told me she could tell what the baby is and asked if I wanted to know. I didn't. I still was convinced I wasn't having a baby and didn't want to bond with it.

I allowed myself feelings of normalcy on vacation in Virginia Beach. While there, I got to spend some time with Barb and Jon and their daughter Rebecca, born on August 1, a few days after Solomon was due. It's difficult not to imagine what life would be like with him there. I endured many uncomfortable moments but worked very hard to conceal them. For me, someone was missing. But all things considered, I actually had an enjoyable vacation. The time with Eric alone was priceless.

As summer began, I was getting large and uncomfortable. My hands started to itch. I thought I might have cholestasis and convinced myself I would lose the baby after thirty seven weeks. I was so upset, I called my OB and he sent me to the hospital, to L&D, to be checked out. And who was attending to me, none other but The Face, the doctor who subtly predicted I would lose Solomon. The last face I wanted to see was his, but surprisingly after I'd been hooked up to the fetal monitor and given blood and given urine and had my blood pressure checked and my hands looked at, the doctor had a different face. He actually smiled when he told me everything looked fine. But when I talked to my OB and he revealed my liver enzymes were elevated, the bubble burst and I was back to square one believing I'll lose the baby.

Eric always treated this as a normal pregnancy. So when I walked up the stairs to Patrick's Pub one Saturday afternoon, I was somewhat surprised to see my family and friends there, yelling "Surprise!" A baby shower for me. I sat in the restaurant among my family and closest friends and let them pamper me. My dad videotaped the whole thing. Even my brother and his wife flew up for this from Atlanta. And for those few hours, I enjoyed being waited on and actually believed my dream would come true.

A few weeks later Eric and I completed Lamaze birthing classes and a CPR class and a baby care class. All that was left for me was a Breastfeeding class and to have the baby, if I was going to have the baby. In the final weeks leading up to Alison's birth, I was seeing my OB every two to three days. I'd be hooked up to the fetal monitor and have a brief sonogram just to make sure everything was fine.

The final weeks were very difficult. My beloved cat, Baby, was dying. We were doing our best to medicate her and for the greater part of nine months she was responding. On August 4th, she gave up her will to live. We knew it was time to release her from the earth. Eric and I took her to the veterinarian's office and she was put to rest. I couldn't stop crying. She was the middle cat of our feline trilogy, and by far she had the sweetest nature. She liked everyone and would have made a great pet for the baby. The grief of losing her on top of the grief of losing Solomon and Baby Z was incredibly huge. I called my OB and he assured me all my crying wouldn't hurt the baby. Lynn, my friend from my loss group and on the SPALS web-ring, called to offer her support.

On the morning of August 14th, I woke up to a beautiful, sunny, summer day. However, I couldn't take another minute of living in fear. I'd reached such a state of grief and anxiety I felt completely crazed. I called my OB and asked if I could be delivered that day. Within an hour, Patty, the nurse called me back and said I was scheduled to deliver at four thirty P.M. I'll never forget her words, "Amy, you're going to be a mommy." I hung up the telephone in disbelief and started to cry.

When I could speak, I called Eric to get the ball rolling. He was home in one hour; we packed up and left for the hospital. He took a bunch of photos of me leaving the house and all the time I was thinking, *Here we go again, another trip to the hospital for nothing.*

The hospital staff was waiting. It was a Tuesday afternoon and no one was scheduled to deliver. It was spooky and quiet on the ward. I was given paperwork to sign and clothes to change into and of course another IV was stuck into me. And I kept thinking, *What is the point of all this?* Even as I was listening to the baby's heartbeat on the fetal monitor I was not convinced I was having this baby. And even while I was having contractions and practicing my breathing I was not convinced I was having this baby.

At seven thirty P.M., I was wheeled into the OB surgical room. So many questions ran through my mind, *How did I get here? What's going to happen now?* I prayed to Solomon to make everything OK.

The spinal went in fairly easily. Eric came in, dressed in scrubs, and sat by my head, behind a screen. I was exhausted from the day, from the months and the pregnancy. I felt pulling, heard my OB talking and then everything went silent for me. And that was when I first heard her.

The moment Alison was born, I was born, too. The sound of her crying freed me from the mental hell I was living in. I could feel the veil of grief being lifted from my eyes. I could feel another part of me leaving, all the fear and the anxiety, as if it just walked out the door. I came alive at the sound of her and the sight of her. She was an eight pound two ounce and nineteen and a half inch bundle of love. In that moment, I was new to the world, too.

I'll never understand why I was chosen to endure such suffering. I know others will never understand why I put myself through so much torment. I do understand sometimes you have to stop asking questions to get to the answers.

ERIC

The Decision

There's a shadow hanging over me.
"Yesterday" written by Paul McCartney

Adecision. No, THE DECISION!!! I DON'T KNOW WHY OR WHEN IT HAPPENED BUT SOMEWHERE, SOMETIME I BECAME THE DECISION MAKER.

It's a blur for me now. I know it happened. I think about it some-times but life and the other children mostly overwhelm it now. I lost a child, Solomon. OK, we lost a child.

My wife Amy still mourns it. We view things differently. I mourn in my own way. As I am told, I'm a realist. I live in today, not tomorrow and not in the yesterdays. I remember yesterdays but more on a memory level, not an emotional level. I try to remember only the good in the past and for-get the bad.

Amy tried to help me with this story and she wrote me a note about the above passage:

There were many more decisions you made, anything you want to include:telling Alex, telling friends, picking a name, deciding how to memo-rialize, deciding when we would try again, deciding if you would come to group counseling, deciding if you would go to individual counseling, decid-ing how or not you would support me, seeing friends, clinging to Alex, attending family things, socializing, how was work for you? Any steps you took in deciding how you would move through this process.

Most of these things I let her decide. I was numb. And she had an opinion and I did not. Telling Alex, my five year old, was just a matter of facts for me. I just needed to explain it so he could understand. But when the moment of truth happened I froze. I couldn't come up with words that would give him the information, but not scare or frighten him. In the end, Amy had to tell him. I got too tongue-tied. He didn't understand at first and that was all right but with others' help he started to comprehend.

Telling friends happened if I spoke to them. I did have to call my family and tell them the outcome of Amy being in the hospital. They knew we were there and some were hurt and saddened deeply.

But the decision of a name, when to try again, and even group counseling was all up to Amy.

Group was interesting. I'm not saying I had completely healed. But in terms of healing Amy and I were continents apart. The stories of the others just brought me further down, not up.

She needed something tangible to start the healing process so I just went with whatever she wanted. I also let Amy choose how soon or long it would take to see friends again. She needed her time and space and I gave it to her. The most powerful thing for me, when there were things to forget about, was to get back to work. And that is what I did. Those at work who knew what was going on were supportive of me.

Experts say the strongest sense to bring back memories is your sense of smell. Being at a hospital with our youngest son for a few days made me remember why I hate hospitals. The last time I saw my father alive he was in a hospital bed. I left him that evening with a big kiss and I never saw or got to speak to him again.

The day Amy and I started to lose Solomon comes in flashes. I remember the look on Amy's face coming out of the bathroom after her water broke. I remember pacing in the ER waiting room. I remember sitting in the examining room. And I remember the look on the resident's face after he examined Amy.

I'm the strong one in our home. I kill the bugs, give the kids the tough medicine and even have to give the cats their medicine. But there are just some things I know I couldn't handle.

For the rest of our lives I will have the guilt of convincing Amy to not hold the twenty week fetus. I thought I would be sick at the sight of it. I looked for second and third opinions that day. Had I made the right choice?

Amy was emotionally unable to make any decision. She left it to me. I asked my father-in-law, I asked her personal doctor. I asked two or three nurses, I even asked God, but knew I would get no answer from him.

So I decided because I was told, "You make the decision." Now I get reminded how Amy wishes she did the opposite. Well that's the past and I can't change it.

I get often from Amy that tone in her voice telling me I let her down by the decision I made. I wanted to remember Solomon by the mind's eye view I had of him not the true appearance of him after his stillbirth. In the end, I saw his pictures along with Amy.

I know it's different for the man.

I didn't carry the child and the connection physically was not there but when I get told I didn't care it bothers me because I did. I cared enough to want to have the child, and in those moments when I'm alone in the car on the way to or from work, a song or statement on the radio can make my eyes tear. I let them flow and I don't try to hold it back.

The Decision!

The house, the car ride, the hospital, the waiting for the medicines to induce Amy. The sea of phone calls and people flowing through the room. I'm not a patient man sometimes. It killed me.

Where did my wife go? I understood, after the loss, that she would grieve eighteen months, and that would have been OK but after we got pregnant again it was the worrying that went on. The daily "what if?" Well, this time it worked out better and Alison was born.

Amy still talks about Solomon's due date; that guess date the doctor gives you so you can plan and set up the office poll. That date disappeared the day he was born alive or not. We don't still talk about Alison's or Adam's due dates because there is an actual date not a projected guess. When Amy starts to speak of his due date I try to redirect the conversation somewhere else.

Decisions need to be made, not only for progress to occur, but also for people to advance. Some decisions can be made without thinking; some take hours. Some take no discussions and others need to be hashed out over and over again. When the moment happened I felt the decision I made was good for all.

A Tale of Two Pregnancies

In three words I can sum up everything I've learned about life: it goes on.
Robert Frost

"It's a girl!!!" Magic words said by Dr. Dave. I had a son, Alex, and I lost a son, Solomon. A girl, Alison, this was something new.

For the prior nine months I lived in paranoia hell from Amy being scared she (Alison) wouldn't show up, no matter what good news we would get from the doctor, sonograms, test results or just praise from people; Amy's constant "waiting for the other shoe to drop" attitude.

Amy had a difficult time with the pregnancy. She believed bad things would happen. With every test, and good and positive outcome, Amy would invent or fixate on something negative. We went for a CVS (chorionic villus sampling) and some genetic testing to try to give her some peace of mind, but this only gave her more reasons to search for information about anything that could go wrong. My wife would turn a sneeze into three days of torturous research on the Internet.

For me it was a pregnancy. The barrage of tests, doctor visits and procedures didn't bother me. They just seemed par for the course. Amy can recall in detail today, years later, what happened and in what order. I only remember specific things if she mentions them or describes them. For me it was life. And life just goes on.

The one thing I always recall is I didn't want to finish the nursery. I would work for an hour and stop for a week. Amy didn't even think I should work that hour on it. It got completed about a week before Alison was born. Contrasting that was I was very excited to help Amy's mom plan the baby shower. Amy wanted nothing to do with it. The day turned out to be a wonderful success. Nine months of hell for the precious moment when Alison was born.

Both mother and daughter were beautiful. Even though Amy had a C-section, the anesthesiologist was nice enough to make sure I saw Alison spring into this world. The only other comments I recall from the OR was the nurse while cleaning Alison saying, "No doubt who the father is here;" Alison looked exactly like me. The faces of Amy's mom and grandmother were wonderful when I went to the waiting room to tell them.

Alison is spirited and happy and giving and beautiful. Mother and child are both lovely. Amy went from grieving woman to caring mother in a moment. Amy would have her moments of grief, but at no time would it interfere with the love and caring for Alison.

"Your son has a penis!" More magic words said by Dr. Dave. And now Adam, the last child. If Solomon lived Adam wouldn't exist; how is that even possible? He is so cute, with his warm smile. Adam's pregnancy was very different. The biggest reason was Amy didn't have time to worry as much because she was taking care of Alison. Good distraction. We went through all the same tests again. Doing this while caring for an infant was harder and easier at the same time.

If you looked at us during Adam's pregnancy, you wouldn't have been able to tell we were scared of all the things that could go wrong. In fact until the six month mark, the pregnancy was smooth and problem-free.

The one special thing that happened to help Amy was she was invited to join a SPALS support group. Along with just the ability to socialize with other adults, she and I got to meet some very special and wonderful people. The first few sessions Amy went by herself, but she finally talked me into coming with her. Actually she wasn't allowed to drive anymore (doctor's orders) so I became the driver. So I had to do something during the meetings. Might as well join in.

She assured me there were other men in the group, and there were. I sat there quietly and realized the group members knew a lot about me and the way I grieved. The first time there, more than one person, when introduced to me, said, "So you're Eric." This convinced me I needed to give my side of the story, not just how Amy saw my behavior.

Now there were three children and two pets, a house, a new job, uncertainty. Life was moving, really moving, and I could see the light at the end of the stressful tunnel.

I never got to know Solomon, his warmth, smile, touch, sound, so how can I miss him? I do, but it's different. I miss him in an imaginary way, because I can only imagine all the things he would be. It's more like daydreaming than reality.

Every person grieves in a different way, always depending on your past life experiences, emotional make up and mental maturity. I have unfortunately seen lots of family death in my life and a lot of it happened when I was young. I guess I have a tough skin for it. It's part of life. I am sad, I realize what happened and then I move on quickly. Some of the stages of grief happen continuously and others take a few hours of thought and they are done. But I always get through it quickly.

I am angered sometimes at how Solomon's loss took some of the joy and love out of Amy permanently. But the children who came after are just so fun, how could I live without them? As individuals, as a pair and as a family, we are perfect with each other.

ROSANNA

A Light for Lucas

Don't say good-bye, just say good night
"Say Good Night" written by Beth Nielsen Chapman

January 6, 2002, my life changed. My husband, Carlos, my two girls, Julia and Victoria and I, had just come back from our vacation. I was on my way to a routine doctor's appointment. I was scheduled for a level II sonogram. I was anxious. It had been a normal pregnancy, no bleeding, no morning sickness, and my blood pressure was fine. Though I had a fever that morning, I didn't reschedule because I wanted to relieve my concerns. I voiced some concerns to the technician, because I really had not felt my baby move. She said, "OK, don't worry. I will check everything out."

As the technician was working on me, I could see her face was very serious. She hadn't put any monitors on. I'd asked her what was going wrong, all she said was, "I'm just finishing with your baby's measurements."

I knew something was wrong. My baby's image was on the screen and there was no movement. My heart was in my throat, I couldn't speak. When the tech was done, she said, "The doctor will be in to talk to you."

It was then I knew I had lost my baby.

The doctor confirmed what I already knew: my baby was gone. I remember screaming, "NO, this can't be," but mostly my memories of that moment are blurred. I was able to ask her if she could tell what the sex of my baby was, but she couldn't.

I barely remember calling Carlos and telling him this horrific news. Each breath was difficult. It was like someone had punched me and I was trying to catch my breath. I'd also called my sister, Josephine, who showed up at the doctor's office and just held me and let me cry. She understood everything I felt because it was on the same day years before she had lost her daughter, Danielle.

When Carlos arrived he took me in his arms and held me tight. He was very strong, thank goodness, because I felt like I was coming apart at the seams.

I remember being at the hospital with a piece of paper in hand. It said fetal demise. Carlos handed it to a nurse; they escorted us in to a labor and delivery room. It is hard to recall how long I was there until it was time to give birth, but there was lots of pain both physically and emotionally.

The nurses at the hospital were very sympathetic and tried to make me as comfortable as possible. When it finally came time to deliver my stillborn baby I remember letting out a screeching cry. The doctor said we had a son.

- My husband and I cried together and he held on to me. I felt so empty inside, and just kept saying this had to be a horrible nightmare.

The doctor had recommended we have an autopsy performed, explaining to us there would be only a fifty percent chance it would find the cause of my son's demise. Carlos and I agreed to it. They also took a lot of blood from me and I had some post-delivery testing. I was told I should have the results in six weeks.

My son was placed in my arms all wrapped up with a hat on; it was time for us to say good-bye. The nurse said we could take as long as we needed. As I looked down at my son, I saw a beautiful baby boy. Even though he was twenty three weeks he looked perfect to us. The hardest thing we ever had to do was say good-bye. We had him blessed by a priest. I couldn't bear to hold him for long. I kissed him and promised to keep him in our hearts forever and named him Lucas.

I turned to Carlos and asked him, "What are we going to say to our children?" Victoria was a little over two and we knew she really wouldn't understand, but Julia was just shy of four and she knew I was having a baby. Carlos said he didn't know but together we would try to explain it to them.

Shortly after I delivered my son a social worker, Margaret, came in to give me some literature on pregnancy loss and to let me know there was a support group if I needed one. I don't remember much of my conversation. I felt so numb; I wanted to be left alone. Carlos wasn't with me at the time she came. He was with our families trying to explain what happened. I didn't feel like seeing anyone, so Carlos talked to our parents and told them to come back in the morning.

I was in the hospital for a few days due to a virus. The day came for me to go home. As I was wheeled downstairs, with no baby in my arms, just a memory box with a piece of hair, a bracelet with his name on it, his hat and blanket, I felt so numb. I didn't know how I was going to function. I still had two girls at home who needed my attention.

Arrangements had to be made for Lucas's burial. My sister made them. She picked the spot where he was going to be laid to rest and it's a beautiful place. I thanked God for my sister; I don't think I could have managed those arrangements without her. It was then I realized the pain she felt five years earlier when she lost her daughter. I kept apologizing to her for really not being there for her, and all she said was, "I didn't expect you to be. How could you possibly have known? I know and that is why I'm here for you."

I knew we had to have a talk with Julia. We didn't have anything pre-pared; we just said the baby in mommy's belly wasn't there anymore. She looked at me and said, "Why did you not love the baby?" and with that I took a deep breath and said, "No, my love, I loved your brother more than anything but God needed him to be in heaven with him." She said OK and went to play.

We decided we would have a gravesite ceremony with family and only close friends. On the day of Lucas's burial, I felt an overwhelming sadness. Carlos and I were at home later in the day with our girls. I felt so cheated; it wasn't supposed to be this way. I asked Carlos if we could take a ride back to the cemetery so I could see if Lucas was laid to rest. We must have been thinking the same thing because he was putting on the girls' shoes as I was asking the question. As we drove up to the cemetery and went by Lucas's gravesite, I was trying so hard not to cry, I didn't want the girls to see me crying.

It was hard for me to express my sadness during the daytime. My daughters needed me, but as soon as the night came and my husband came home I went in our room and cried. It was then I decided to call Margaret and ask when her next support group was meeting.

She said her co-worker Monica would be starting a group the following week. I spoke to my husband. He was a little reluctant to go and express his feelings with strangers, but it was something I felt I needed and we decided to go.

The night came for our first of six bereavement sessions. Seeing everyone there was difficult. When it came time to tell our story, I remember trying so hard not to cry but that was impossible. It was there Carlos really opened up and where we began to really heal. Carlos had felt if we never went on vacation then maybe we would have our son today, and I told him I didn't blame him for what happened just as he didn't blame me. The support group not only helped us hea,l but it was there I formed a wonderful friendship with another couple, Lou and Tara. Under unfortunate circumstances we formed a close bond.

Hearing everyone's story I remember a lot of crying and lot of anger and saying, "Oh my God, look at all these couples going through what we are going through." By the time the last session came I had the report on Lucas's autopsy and the tests that were done on me. When it was our time to share I let everyone know the autopsy was inconclusive and my tests showed no abnormalities.

I still had no answer as to why my son died, but I knew it wasn't anything I had done or failed to do. I can't say it made my healing process go any quicker but I had some closure. The friendships with this group helped me get through my next pregnancy in which I birthed a beautiful, healthy baby boy.

It has taken me a long time to accept what happened with Lucas. I read a few books on loss which helped my healing process. I didn't write in a journal, which was recommended; I simply couldn't. Reading helped me; going to the memorial service held at the hospital where I delivered helped me tremendously.

Carlos helped me heal by letting me express myself at any given time. He never told me to 'get over it.' He just let me do what I needed to do to get through a day. I also found solace by attending reunion groups and sharing my story with others and letting them know they aren't alone.

My pain of losing Lucas isn't as sharp as it was two years ago, but it's still there. I endured a lot of sleepless nights. It wasn't until one night I believed Lucas gave me a sign to let me know he was all right. I went to bed and remember being awakened by a kiss. My husband and two children were asleep. I remember feeling a little sigh of happiness. It was then I knew Lucas was watching over us and he was fine. There isn't a day I don't think of him.

Since the day I came home from the hospital Carlos and I wanted to do something to make him a part of our everyday life, so we bought a small angel statue and a small candle. The statue and candle are in our room and every night we light his candle, let it burn for a while, and before we go to sleep one of us blows it out, and we all say goodnight to him. For us it just feels right.

One Magical Night

A whole new world, a dazzling place I never knew.
Let me share this whole new world with you.
"A Whole New World" written by Tim Rice

The day came when I approached my husband and said I would like to have another baby. He said, "Are you sure?" He asked me because we had tried a few months prior and I'd miscarried at six weeks. I was devastated and told Carlos, "No more."

I didn't have a good experience at the hospital that had performed my D&C. The staff kept shuffling me around from floor to floor. I was on a gurney waiting in the hallway until someone could figure out where to put me. I felt like screaming, "You idiots! I'm here for a D&C. Find my doctor and let's get this night over with so I can go home." I just kept thinking, *When will this nightmare be over?*

Finally someone came to my rescue, a very lovely nurse who put me in labor and delivery at the very far end of the ward until my doctor was ready. At last the D&C was over and home we went. I was numb all over again and the feelings of losing Lucas seemed so fresh and vivid.

At my follow-up appointment my doctor said one loss had nothing to do with the other, and if I wanted to try again to get pregnant to wait one month and that he was really sorry for what had happened.

It was approximately nine months since I lost Lucas and we were getting ready to go on a family vacation to Disney World, the first family vacation since we lost Lucas. We went away in October rather than over Christmas. I wasn't ready to go back to St. Thomas where we had been before; I wanted to go someplace new. We had a wonderful time; it was just what we needed to help us deal with the losses.

I guess they call Disney a magical place where dreams can come true for a reason. A month after we came back I found out I was pregnant. I was a little surprised because Carlos and I discussed trying again before we left and decided if it happened over the vacation it would be great, but we would go really to enjoy ourselves and would concentrate on having another baby when we came home.

I didn't tell my family immediately. However I told Carlos on the telephone I thought I was pregnant and was going out to buy a pregnancy test. He wanted me to wait until he got home but the box just kept on staring at me, and I had to take the test. It was positive and I immediately called Carlos. He was a little disappointed I didn't wait for him but he understood I needed to know. I opted to wait until I was eight weeks along before seeing my OB so there would be no doubt I was pregnant. I wanted to be able to see on the sonogram machine a beating heart. I took a pregnancy test once a week until the day of my appointment.

Carlos and I were both nervous; the nurse in the office knew of my situation and took us right in.

The machine was on but with the sound turned off. The doctor was examining me and when he turned the monitor toward me, the nurse turned on the volume. It was the most beautiful sound, my baby's heart beating. It was like a weight had been lifted and I could breathe a little bit better. Though I could have chosen to come back in two weeks, I opted for one month. I didn't want to stress over this pregnancy, I knew it would be difficult anyway.

I continued with my monthly visits and couldn't wait until fifteen weeks when I could hear the baby's heartbeat with the Doppler. Carlos and I decided against getting the home monitor for me to listen at home, just on the off chance I got a dud, or I wasn't using it correctly. I already felt uptight and didn't want to add more stress and have my girls get my backlash. I wasn't ready to face another disappointment.

I didn't start going to a support group when I first learned I was pregnant again, but when I got home from my fifteen week appointment I called Anna, the social worker from the bereavement group, and asked her when her next meeting for SPALS was taking place. I was reluctant to go because it was on the first anniversary of Lucas's death.

It turned out this group was what I needed to keep some of my sanity through the next few months. I also went by myself, it was something I needed to do and something Carlos didn't need.

It was time to tell family and friends of our good news. We decided the first to know should be our girls. They took the news very well. Victoria was very excited and Julia seemed a little nervous, but I assured her everything was fine and the doctor was taking good care of me. That seemed to ease her mind; she gave me a big smile and said she wanted to have a brother.

The two people I had not yet told were Tara and Lou, good friends from the support group. I knew Tara was still trying to get pregnant, she wanted to have another baby.

We decided to take them out to dinner. I was a little nervous, and wore a heavy sweater so I wouldn't give anything away before its time. They were very happy for us. The tears we cried were both tears of joy, for us, and tears of sadness for Tara and Lou.

The day came for my level II sonogram. I wasn't nervous about finding out if the baby was alive. It must have known I needed a lot of reassurance-kicking. I was nervous about it being healthy. We opted not to do an amnio-centesis.

The sonogram technician came in and started taking measurements and the sound was on the whole time and the baby's heartbeat was very strong. Carlos and I decided not to find out the sex of the baby and to wait for the delivery. Everything looked good, another stage successfully completed!

At my SPALS meeting I told everyone the good news. With each passing week, as I got closer to my delivery, the friends I made there became a more important tool for me to get through my pregnancy. I felt so very comfortable with everyone. In between my meetings if I needed to express myself I would e-mail the group. This helped me so much.

As I approached my thirty-eighth week I discussed induction with my doctor and he told me the hospital wouldn't allow any inductions unless medically necessary, but if I wanted to, I could go the hospital where I had had my D&C. Out of the question! I said I would wait with baited breath and I did.

On June 30th, I started to feel some light contractions. Again my OB suggested I go to the D&C hospital since he was in a meeting, but I insisted I was going to Winthrop and asked him to call over there to let them know I'd be arriving. I never wanted to go to the D&C hospital again. Having lost Lucas and then being subjected to such an ordeal with my D&C, the last place I wanted to deliver was there.

We arrived at the Winthrop. I knew Margaret, the social worker and one of the SPALS group leaders, was on call so I asked the nurse to please let her know I had arrived.

We met the on-call doctor. I called my sister Josephine and through her sister-in-law (who worked at the hospital) I was reassured this doctor was excellent and I remember thinking my angel Lucas was looking out for us all along. I hung up the telephone and said to Carlos, "Let's bring our baby into the world."

The doctor checked and told me it is time to push. We heard the baby cry, and the doctor pronounced, "You have a son."

He placed him on my stomach. Carlos and I were in shock, tears of joy for our son, Antonio, and tears of sadness for Lucas.

The wait was over and the phone-call chain began, letting our family and friends know we delivered a healthy baby boy. We looked at him and both agreed he looked like our older daughter, Julia, whereas Lucas resembled our younger daughter, Victoria. As soon as I was in a hospital room, Carlos's parents came with our girls and we introduced them to their new brother. They were so excited and the smiles were priceless.

We still light a candle for Lucas every night, and when we blow out his candle we tell him goodnight and that we love him.

LYNN M

Losing Kailyn Nicole

I can see your star, shining down on me
"Together Again" written by Janet Jackson, James Harris III, Terry Lewis
and René Elizondo, Jr.

We celebrated our fourth wedding anniversary in September, 2003.

Four years ago I was in such a different place, and I never thought I would be where I am today. Although my wedding anniversary is a celebration of my marriage with Sean, he wouldn't be my husband if it weren't for our daughter. My wedding anniversary is a reminder of my past that we worked through and battled to find our place in this world again.

In June 1999, I found out I was pregnant. Sean and I were not married. There was no question of my choice during the pregnancy test of what I was going to do. I didn't know how Sean would take it; whether he would stick by me or leave me.

When I told him he was very excited, and scared. He took it much better than my family. I think the hardest part was finding the right time to tell them.

My mom was at my house one day, filleting chicken cutlets, telling me a story about my older brother and his girlfriend. They had been having problems and mom said, "She should just get pregnant so they can get married." So in turn, I said, "Ha, funny you should mention that, 'cause I'm pregnant."

I felt like I was in that Molly Ringwald movie *For Keeps*, "I'm pregnant, can you pass the potatoes?" It didn't go over as well as I thought. She swung that knife around yelling and asked me, "What were you thinking?" After a while she calmed down, we told her we had thought very hard about our decision and we were keeping the baby.

We decided to get married. I'd always wanted a big wedding, with the poofy white dress and many bridesmaids. On September 18 we vowed to love one another until death do us part.

I was twenty weeks along at the time. Although I'm not sure how many people knew I was pregnant, I did look like a princess. You couldn't even tell I was pregnant. People later on told me I was one of the most beautiful brides they had ever seen. We had a great reception; everyone had so much fun. The future looked so bright. We spent a couple of days in Newport, RI, as our honeymoon. We even purchased a nightlight for the baby. It was a frog light that when lit up would circle the room. I couldn't wait to use it.

My pregnancy was completely uneventful. I went to my monthly checkups, had all the usual tests, and sonograms. The baby was growing well. We didn't find out the sex of the baby since we wanted to be surprised.

At thirty six weeks, I noticed some spotting; The doctor sent me for a sonogram, and that confirmed my baby was breech. Not a big deal, they said, either the baby will flip or a C-section will be performed. I can still remember the days following the sonogram, feeling the baby push its hands up. During this time it felt like I already had a relationship with it. Even through she or he was still in my stomach, we were already playing Mommy–Baby games.

February 13, 2000 was my baby shower. It was supposed to be a surprise but I had a feeling what was going on. I received so many gifts, and all these beautiful little outfits. The next day I felt terribly ill. I didn't get off the couch the entire day. It felt like I was coming down with the flu.

Tuesday I felt better, and Wednesday I mentioned to my mom I hadn't really felt the baby move much. Ironically, with those words I had a Braxton-Hicks contraction and you could see the baby move. Thursday morning was my routine thirty eight week check-up. On the drive to the office, I turned to my husband and said, "If there is no heartbeat you will have to commit me."

I was beyond scared; it was as if I already knew — women's intuition.

As I lay on the table, the doctor put the Doppler up to my belly. I didn't hear a heartbeat. The doctor kept moving the Doppler around, still nothing. It was getting even scarier for me because the baby was breech, the heartbeat had been in the same position for a couple of weeks; and he still couldn't find it. He said he would be right back. He came back into the room, said, "Let's do a sonogram." Once they put the wand to my belly, they pointed to the monitor and said, "See, that's where it should be and there isn't anything." My doctor grabbed my hand, and said, "I'm so sorry, sweetie, there is no heartbeat."

I didn't cry, I didn't do anything. He left and got my husband, who came in looking grayer than gray. We just hugged, and I kept repeating over and over I couldn't believe this was happening. They told us to go straight over to the hospital, a five minute drive. It seemed like forever to get there.

Once there, they brought in the sonogram machine, (let me tell you how much I hate those machines even to this day), and again confirmed there was indeed no heartbeat. I still didn't cry, just kept repeating over and over, "OH, MY GOD."

Sean called our moms; I'd told him not to tell them what was going on, just to come straight to the hospital. Within hours, both families were at our sides. Everyone was crying and hugging. I'll never forget, my oldest brother coming in and holding me so tight.

They induced me right away, and my water broke after a few hours. Twenty six hours later on February 18 at two fourteen P.M., Kailyn Nicole silently entered this world. She weighed six pounds, one ounce and was nineteen inches.

The staff took her out of the room and cleaned her up and brought her back in, dressed in a pretty little dress with a white knit hat. She was swaddled in a baby blanket. Sean wouldn't hold her, but I knew I couldn't go on if I didn't. I looked her over, took the blanket off of her and checked her out. She was perfect. My perfect baby daughter.

We held her for a while and said our goodbyes, and I cried as I had never cried before. I stayed in the hospital until Sunday. They told me I could leave at any point, but I was afraid to go home. All of Kailyn's stuff was there, waiting for her. I didn't want to face that.

My family made funeral arrangements. She was buried in a baby cemetery close to our house. Our family and close friends came for support, about thirty people, more than I ever thought would come.

We had a luncheon thrown by my best friend's family. Going home afterwards was tougher than I ever could have imagined. As I was sitting at my best friend's table looking around at who was left, I knew I had to go home. I just didn't want to. I knew I couldn't stay there forever, but at that time, it would have been OK if I did. I eventually got myself together and left.

Everything was still set up for Kailyn. As much as my family wanted to help me, I'd told everyone not to touch anything. I would put her things away myself. We left things the way they were for a couple of days.

In the middle of March, I went to Cancun with my family, as I needed to get away. Sean didn't want to go. He thought it better to throw himself into his work, but I was still on maternity leave. I lay on the beach and did nothing for a whole week. It was great just to lie there.

When I returned from vacation, I met with my doctor, who informed me Kailyn's death was a fluke. She had died from a cord accident. It was wrapped seven times around her neck. A true knot was also found in the cord. He informed me I would be watched over more closely next time around.

My hospital's social work department contacted me. They were in the process of starting a new bereavement group and asked if I would be interested. I definitely was.

The group consisted of four couples: one had a few miscarriages after a successful pregnancy, the second lost a baby midway through, and another lost twins. It was a place to just let it all out. Sean didn't want to be there, but he went and supported me. Sometimes it pissed me off, because he wouldn't say a word, and here was I pouring my heart out to these people who I didn't know.

After group ended in June, we adopted our dog, Dillon, from North Shore Animal League, a few months after losing Kailyn. He was three months old, his birthday sometime in March, the original month Kailyn was due. We had discussed getting a dog for a while.

We went to the shelter and we saw this cute little puppy asleep in his crate. Sean wanted to take him out and play, but I kept telling him to look at the size of those paws. I gave in and went into the play room with the dog, where we tossed the ball a couple of times, saying he was going be huge. The deciding factor was when Dillon went to retrieve a ball; he came back and laid down right between Sean's legs. I looked at the girl who worked there and said "OK, give me an application, we're taking him home." He was our 'baby' and to this day still is, even though he's 125 pounds and Aidan can ride him as a pony.

Aidan's Arrival

I knew I loved you before I met you
"I Knew I Loved You" written by Darren Hayes and Darren Jones

It took me thirteen months to conceive again. I was taking my temperature, charting, taking those ovulation test kits, but nothing happened. Everyone kept telling me to relax, it would happen when my body is ready. Yeah right! Like I wanted to hear that. I wanted it to happen *now*. My doctor sent me for a hysterosalpingogram, to make sure there were no blockages, but there was one. The dye wouldn't go through my right Fallopian tube. I was scheduled for a laparoscopy.

They found my right ovary isn't connected to the fallopian tube, it's a birth defect and it cannot be corrected. So basically I can only get pregnant when I ovulate on my left side. Kailyn was a complete surprise, pretty much a miracle in getting pregnant and here I was struggling to conceive again.

Finally in April, I learned I conceived my son. I was on a business trip in Houston, in my hotel room enjoying a cup of coffee with my co-workers, recuperating from a night out. I got up to go to the bathroom before we left for our meeting, and I noticed some spotting when I wiped. I came out of the bathroom, and said, "Either I'm getting my period or I'm pregnant." Both my co-workers were so excited; they had known I'd been trying for so long. They insisted we go to the drug store for an early pregnancy test. I agreed.

We bought the test, arrived at our meeting and I excused myself to go to the bathroom. I took the test and was amazed to see the faintest second line appear. I was done for the day. I don't remember a single thing about any of the meetings I was in. I was floating on cloud nine.

I called my doctor and informed him I saw the second line but I was spotting. He wanted me off my feet. I explained I was in Texas, but I would try my hardest and would see him the following Monday. We left the next morning and I remained on the couch at home until Monday when I saw my doctor and blood-work confirmed I was indeed pregnant again. FINAL-LY!

My pregnancy this time around was very different. My doctor and a perinatologist saw me every three weeks in my first trimester. I was spotting constantly. At thirteen weeks, I ended up in the hospital for unexplained bleeding. I was put on bed rest for several weeks. I bought one of those Baby-Beat® Doppler machines to listen for the baby's heartbeat, it never left my side. If I went out for dinner with friends, it was in my pocketbook. I listened at least twice a day to the baby's heartbeat. People probably thought I was crazy, but for me it was peace of mind.

I also joined an Internet group for women who have gone through a loss and are pregnant again. There are over 400 women on the list. Some were going through their SPALS pregnancy, some were trying to get pregnant, and some were still waiting to try to get pregnant.

At twenty weeks, we found out during a level II sonogram we were having a boy. My initial feeling was a little disappointment. I really wanted a girl. That feeling lasted only a quick moment, and then reality set in. A healthy, living, breathing baby is what I wanted, the sex didn't matter. I was told all looked fine and I could return to work part-time.

From twenty eight weeks on I had Non-Stress tests and Bio Physical Profile tests twice a week. I was sent several times to L&D at the hospital for evaluations. The staff started to know me by my first name. Since my daughter died at thirty eight and a half weeks, I would have an amniocentesis at thirty seven weeks. If this baby's lungs were mature they would do a C-section the next day.

December 4th I went for my amniocentesis and at five P.M. was notified by my doctor the baby's lungs were mature enough. YIPPIE! We decided Thursday would be his birthday.

Wednesday I pampered myself. I went to the nail salon and got a manicure and pedicure. I didn't really set too much up for fear we wouldn't bring our new baby home. The only thing we had out was the bassinet and a few clothes. I didn't want to go through what I had gone through with my daughter.

I don't think I slept more than two hours. We left our house at seven A.M.; I made sure my Doppler was with me. The entire ride to the hospital I kept checking his heartbeat.

In pre-op I was hooked up to the monitor. My mom came and stayed with us until it was time for the C-section.

I was brought into the operating room, and given a spinal anesthetic. Sean came in shortly. Surgery started. I remember saying, "Does anyone smell that?" and no one answered. It was the laser making the first incision.

At ten forty A.M. Aidan Michael arrived in this world, weighing in at seven pounds, twelve ounces and nineteen inches long. He started screaming right away. The doctor held him over the curtain for us to see, instantly I started crying. What a wonderful sound, I never wanted it to end.

Once I was stitched back up I was rolled over to see him quickly. He looked just like Kailyn. He had her long eyelashes, long legs. Aidan's hair was darker though. Even though he was crying well, he had wet lungs. He was taken into the NICU for oxygen. He was breathing on his own, but needed some help. Sean went with the staff and I was taken to recovery.

I didn't get to hold Aidan until later in the evening. We went to the NICU and I didn't want to leave. I just wanted to hold him forever. I remember telling the doctor when he came in to check on me, "You better find a reason for me not to be able to leave, because I'm not leaving without my baby this time."

Aidan was in the NICU until Saturday morning. We were released together on Monday and left the hospital as a family. What a moment, I was finally leaving with a living, breathing, healthy baby. It was a beautiful thing.

Aidan is now a healthy two-year-old. I look at him and wonder, *Would his sister have done the same things*? When my son grows up he will know he has a sister in heaven; that she was very much wanted, very much loved, and missed everyday. I take him to the cemetery and when we are ready to leave I always say, "Give baby Kailyn a kiss, and say bye-bye." It's so sweet; he blows a kiss in the air and says, "bye-bye."

I'm currently trying for my second SPALS baby. I've been trying to get pregnant for eleven months. My regular OB recommended a fertility specialist. I've had two Intrauterine Inseminations (IUI) and am currently waiting for my next. This experience is still as frustrating as it was when I was trying for Aidan. I'm hoping I can have a normal pregnancy and maybe enjoy this one like I enjoyed being pregnant with Kailyn. It seems that with a SPALS pregnancy there is no such thing as normal pregnancy anymore.

Even though the tragedy of my daughter was four years ago, there isn't a day I don't think of her and what could have been. I question everything.

I look at my son, my husband. I look at my house, *How would this be different*? I know I'm not a bad person and I didn't deserve my daughter to die. No one does. But it happened and I learned with the help of women who understand, a great family and great friends, you can get through everything. One day I know I will meet my daughter. I'm OK living my life the way it's supposed to be until then. Sometimes, faith is the only way to go.

LINDA

Our Beloved Daughter, Sarah Ann

*Nobody realizes the inner strength they have
until they have to pick themselves up by heartstrings.*
Author Unknown

John and I were married March 20, 1999 and knew we wanted to have a family. We waited awhile before we decided when it was time. March 21, 2002, we found out we were pregnant with our first child. We were thrilled beyond words and worried, as anyone would be.

My pregnancy was normal, even the morning sickness that accompanied it for the first four months. We didn't find out what we were having, a boy or a girl, because it didn't matter. We wanted a healthy, beautiful child. I remember going through my pregnancy with elation and wonderment at who our child would look like, what traits it would have from each of us and what our new life would be like. We were choosing names and planning our baby's future.

We made it through the first three months, which everyone always said were the most critical and after that you would be fine. Like many others, we were so naive.

John and I were so happy the baby would be born near Thanksgiving, John's favorite holiday. We would have such a wonderful Christmas. No present could be better than the gift of a child. Our family gave us a beautiful shower and we received everything we needed. Now it was just waiting for the birth of our child.

Time marched on and we had our level II sonogram to check all of the organs and measurements. Everything checked out fine. The due date was November 30th.

The baby was very active all the time. I remember thinking the baby would come out running a marathon. I never had to worry about doing the kick count sheet, since the baby never really stopped moving, which later would prove fatal. In my thirty-sixth week, I recall the baby had the hiccups four to six times a day and I thought it was odd. I know people told me their baby also had the hiccups in utero. I told my doctor about it and he said it was normal, so I went on thinking so.

November 30th came and went and I was very anxious. I'd said from the beginning I didn't want to go past my due date and had expressed that to my doctor and he said with a first pregnancy, it could go two weeks either way. I wasn't happy with his response.

As each day went by, I was more and more nervous. I felt something was going to happen. Then December 3rd came. It was around eleven P.M. and I started to have what I thought were contractions. They lasted about an hour and then stopped and I fell asleep. I awoke at five A.M. and had to go to the bathroom. I remember waking and not feeling the baby move, which was very strange. I even ate several spoonfuls of sugar to see if the baby would move and nothing happened. I went to the bathroom and I wiped and there was an abnormal color discharge and I panicked. I called my doctor and from what I described he said it seemed fine, but to meet him at the hospital anyway. We drove to the hospital and the whole time I knew it wasn't good.

When we arrived, the nurse hooked me up to the fetal monitor and was searching for the heartbeat, which never had to be looked for in the past. The nurse had always been able to find it immediately. After a few minutes, she called in another nurse and the outcome was the same. Our baby's heart had stopped.

I became hysterical. I remember thinking my worst nightmare came true. During the middle of my pregnancy I read a story about a woman whose baby died due to the cord being wrapped around the neck. At my next doctor's appointment I asked him about that and he said the chances of it happening were slim to none, but I had the fear from then on. It turned out our beautiful daughter, Sarah Ann, died due to cord entanglement. The cord was abnormal, three times the length of a normal cord and didn't have the protective coating of Wharton's Jelly on it. This made the cord extremely flexible and easy for the baby to become entangled.

The forty eight hours following the news our daughter was gone were the worst time John and I had ever experienced.

A social worker came to talk about what had happened and what would happen. I remember her asking us if we wanted to see the baby after it was born and I couldn't conceive of doing that. I thought, *The baby is dead, why would I want to see it*?

I'm glad she and the nurses continued to talk to us through the labor because we changed our minds and agreed we wanted to see and hold the baby. That proved to be one of the most important decisions we made. As hard as it was, I couldn't imagine how I would have felt if I hadn't seen her. I would have regretted it forever.

Even though I was four days past my due date, I wasn't dilated at all. The doctor started me on an internal cervix softener and after twelve hours I only dilated two centimeters. They administered another dose and things started to progress.

I was having contractions which were extremely painful, so I requested an epidural. That was the first of three separate epidural lines they had to insert. The doctor who began the epidural couldn't seem to get it in the right spot and I felt ninety percent of my labor. It got to the point where they had to give me a sedative. I slept for three hours and then it started again. Finally, there was a shift change and another doctor came in and inserted another line and it worked immediately. Thank goodness for that doctor.

After more than thirty hours of labor, our angel was born. What got me through was thinking all of these doctors are wrong and she would be fine.

It was then we found out it was a girl and since we planned to name a daughter Sarah Ann before this happened, that's the name we gave her. I didn't feel I would be able to give her another name and also wouldn't be able to use Sarah Ann in the future. That name belonged to her. Sarah Ann was born at one twenty-seven P.M. weighing eight pounds six ounces. She was twenty two inches long.

After the birth, they took Sarah into another room, cleaned her up and put her in a pretty little white and purple dress. About a half hour later they brought her to us and we just crumbled. She was so beautiful with a head of dark curly hair, my nose and my husband's hands and toes. I wanted so badly for her to open her eyes and start crying. She didn't.

We held her for an hour. My sister, mother-in-law, father-in-law and brother-in-law were there also and held her. My parents were at home with my sister's children. The nurse took Sarah Ann away and that was the first and last time we held our baby girl. If I'd known what I know now, I would have held her longer and asked to bathe and change her.

We received a memory box from the hospital with her footprints, ID bracelet, a little memory book the nurses filled out and a certificate of Baptism, which the nurses performed. The priest we called for wouldn't perform any type of Baptism since the baby was already gone. He said the Catholic religion doesn't do that since a baby goes straight to heaven anyway.

We left the hospital the next morning. I couldn't wait to get out of there. You cannot imagine the feeling of leaving the hospital without the child you just spent so many hours delivering. We drove home in silence, except for the sobbing. When we walked into our home, I fell to my knees and couldn't believe I wasn't carrying my baby into her home. Her nursery was all done and the door remained closed for a long time. Even the Christmas tree was there, waiting for her.

My wonderful husband made all of the arrangements to lay our child to rest. I couldn't bear the thought of doing it. We decided we were just

going to have a graveside ceremony. Long-time friends of my parents oper-
ated the funeral home we chose, and they were beyond wonderful. They
dressed Sarah Ann in her beautiful pink coming-home outfit my mother
bought, and with a hand knitted pink blanket and hat made by my mother.
Since my parents were unable to come to the hospital to see Sarah Ann, they
went with us to see her at the funeral home. I wanted to see her again so
badly. We brought one of our wedding pictures and I wrote her a note on
the back and left it with her. I also gave her the gold cross necklace I wore
almost everyday of my pregnancy with her. I wanted her to have something
from me.

One of the more intense moments was when my mother saw Sarah for
the first time, in the coffin. In retrospect, I think this was a bad way for my
mother to see her. It would have been better if mom hadn't seen her in such
a devastating environment. My father was unable to bring himself to see
her, which I was fine with. I found out my father's sister also had a stillbirth
many years ago and he was there to help her and it devastated him. I cannot imagine what he felt, this happened to his daughter also. We said our
final goodbyes and left the funeral home and our beautiful daughter. I wish
I'd asked to hold her one more time.

The ceremony was on Monday, December 9th. It was short and I don't
really remember most of it. After the service, everyone came back to our
house. It got to the point I needed to take something to mellow and I took a
Valium.

The days and weeks after losing Sarah were unbelievable. To this day
I'm still angered and bewildered as to why this happened to us. We wanted
this child so much and there are people out in the world who have children
who don't deserve them and also people who harm and kill their children.
Why would God do this to a family who wants a child?

One of the biggest challenges for me was to get over the fact I thought
they buried my child alive and she was trying to get out. I kept going back
to the cemetery and at one point I wanted to dig her up to make sure she

was gone. I also wanted to just crawl right in next to her because I couldn't imagine the pain ever going away. People say it gets easier. I'm here to tell you it doesn't. I still feel the pain as I did when it happened. My heart is just broken in a way that can never be repaired.

We reached out for counseling because we knew we needed it. The first group we attended was through a local church and was open-ended and we still go to the meetings, which are held once a month. The second group was through our hospital, which was a six week program. Both proved to be invaluable to John and me. It was a place to go where we could talk about our child and not feel like we were making anyone uncomfortable. I already know what one of Sarah's purposes was. She has brought to us many new friends who will be friends for life. We have formed such very close friendships with several other couples, I couldn't imagine not having them in our lives. I feel I've known them all my life. Our children are the reason we all became friends. Although, I wish I'd never met any of them and we would all have our beautiful children.

My doctor wanted to do a complete work-up on me and sent me for every blood test imaginable. They took twenty six vials of blood from me to perform many different tests. Although it isn't life threatening and it may or may not have played a role in Sarah's death, I was found to have MTHFR mutation, a clotting disorder. After my doctor received the results, he wanted me to meet with a specialist. The specialist went over my entire record and agreed the cause of death was cord-related. He explained the many different types of clotting disorders. He, and my doctor, said in any future pregnancy, the treatment for this would be a baby aspirin and an additional milligram of folic acid everyday.

Through all of this, I started researching stillbirths and clotting disorders on the Internet and found some very disturbing information. Although clotting disorders are apparently very common, they aren't part of a regular screen when you become pregnant. What I also found extremely disturbing is that there are about ten times more stillbirths in a year than there are SIDS deaths, yet very little or no research has been done and there is no federal funding at all to support any research. I'm not stating there shouldn't be a focus on SIDS and the research isn't needed, however, a comparable effort should be made with research and prevention of stillbirths.

One of the most comprehensive websites I found attributed to stillbirths is www.stillnomore.org. This website was created by Richard Olsen, who lost his daughter, Camille, to stillbirth in August 2000. He is the founder of the National Stillbirth Society and has made tremendous strides in many different areas regarding stillbirth. As all of us who have experienced a stillbirth know, you just cannot find enough information out there. Richard is committed to bringing all of these issues into the public eye. I found part of the problem with stillbirths is nobody ever wants to discuss it because it is an extremely disturbing subject. People should just imagine how disturbing it is for the parents. So much that needs to be done in order to combat this horrible tragedy.

Through the months following Sarah's passing, I became obsessed with having a child. I thought Sarah was my only chance of having a baby. I asked my doctor when I could start trying again and he gave me the go ahead after my six week check up. He said after six weeks, your uterus goes back to normal and there is no reason why you cannot try immediately. That was all I needed to hear.

After the first month I found I wasn't pregnant, I was devastated. I did everything the books say to predict when you ovulate, and was also using the ovulation kits. I thought we had nailed it and it didn't work. This confirmed my fear of not having another baby. Month two came and to my surprise, after three pregnancy tests and two blood tests, we were pregnant again. It was March 17, 2003, just one week earlier than when we found out we were pregnant with Sarah the year before. This put the due date as November 25th and Sarah's due date was November 30th.

Little Brother, Jack Peter

Count your blessings, not your burdens.
Author Unknown

When you become pregnant for the first time, you go through your pregnancy almost with blinders on. Millions of women have babies and there's no reason to think you will not. You think of all of the things you will do with your child, what they will be, all of the "firsts," choosing names and planning your life with them.

This is what normal expectant mothers do, not ones who experience a stillbirth. Mothers who experience a stillbirth go through a subsequent pregnancy with the thought this baby will also die. My fear for thirty seven weeks.

My doctor was very understanding and accommodating. He said whatever I needed, he would do. I bet to this day, he wishes he had never said those words. I was beyond neurotic.

When I first found out I was pregnant, I showed up at my doctor's office at seven thirty A.M. for the first blood test. He said he would put a rush on it and would call me back that day. The hours passed and I didn't hear from him and I thought it could only be bad news. At ten P.M., out of my mind, I paged him and luckily he was still in the office. He checked and said the test came back positive and he wanted to see me again the next day for another blood test to ensure the HCG levels were going up. I did as he said and everything was fine. This was only the beginning of what I consider to be nine months of mental hell for John and me.

It's hard to put into words what my mental state was during this pregnancy. I felt as if I was another person living a very troubled person's life. Every minute of every day I worried I was going to lose this baby. I had some morning sickness for the first three months, but it wasn't anything compared to what I experienced with Sarah. I thought since I wasn't as sick, this wasn't going to be a successful pregnancy. I started thinking the pregnancy was different because I wasn't having a girl, I was having a boy. This is before we found out the gender.

At no time was another pregnancy a method to try and replace Sarah. We wanted to have a child. Most women who have gone through losing a child may think about replacement, but do not say it. I had difficulty dealing with the fact we might not have a girl. Even though we didn't find out with Sarah what gender we were having, I knew it was a girl. I just felt it. I was hoping for another since my niece was going to be two and I thought it would be great to have a little girl and they would grow up and be best friends. Regardless, I would have loved either.

My level II sonogram came along and we decided we wouldn't find out what we were having. According to the technician, everything was fine and we were right on schedule.

Three weeks later, we received a call from my doctor; he wanted me to have another sonogram since he wasn't able to clearly make out the baby's face and back of the head. This sent me into a tailspin. I immediately went to his office and, of course, made him do a regular sonogram to confirm the baby was still alive, and then went on a tangent about how it could take so long to figure out I needed another sonogram.

Apparently, he wasn't made aware of it when the original paperwork arrived. I then thought there was something else he wasn't telling me and he wanted to see another sonogram to confirm bad news.

I called the lab to schedule another sonogram. I told them I would be in the office in an hour and wouldn't leave until it had been done. Once I arrived, I informed them of my situation and they took me immediately. I was lying on the table crying and John was with me. I turned to him and said I needed to know what we were having and he agreed.

The technician had no problem determining it was a boy. I burst into tears. It wasn't because I wasn't happy it was a boy, it was just that, this is the first time I'm admitting this, I wanted a girl. Not to replace Sarah, but to have what I lost. It took me awhile to realize the fact we were having a boy and I'm glad we found out when we did. Knowing how I reacted and just the stress of the following four months and the delivery, I was able to focus on those things and not wonder how I would react when the baby was born. The results of the second sonogram were faxed to my doctor and, of course, everything was fine.

When I first met with my doctor, he listed tests we would be doing this time, including a Biophysical Profile and the Non Stress Test starting at twenty six weeks and every two weeks after. When I hit my twenty-fourth week, I reminded him of this and he said we could start it at thirty one weeks. I think you know what happened next. On the day I began my twenty-sixth week, I started with the BPPs and NSTs. I was seeing my doctor every two weeks and having the BPP every two weeks, therefore, I was getting checked every week.

This seemed too long for me, so I maintained the once a week visits with an occasional freak-out here and there. I, not my doctor, am fortunate I work right down the street from his office. So, whenever I had one of my little episodes, I was at his office in five minutes. Of course, the major concern I had every time I went for the BPP was where the cord was. They couldn't do a thing about it if it was around the neck, but I needed to know. Every visit they would do a Doppler sonogram of the cord and the blood flow was always perfect and the cord wasn't around the baby's neck at anytime.

The baby was very active, which made me nervous thinking he was wrapping himself in the cord. It also didn't help whenever I didn't feel him move for a short period of time, I would eat anything with sugar to get him moving.

I realize this wasn't a good thing to do, but if I didn't, I would have been living at my doctor's office. I wanted to get a home Doppler machine, but continued to talk myself out of it since I wasn't proficient with its use and would probably cause my husband and myself more anxiety than what we were already going through.

John came with me to every visit because I was terrified at one of the visits they would tell me they couldn't find the heartbeat and I would be alone. When I was pregnant with Sarah, I went to the routine doctor visits and didn't have anything extra going on. Not this time.

Throughout this pregnancy, John and I attended bi-weekly SPALS group sessions at the hospital. It was helpful to attend these meetings and talk with others going through the same issues. It helped with the fact we were still grieving the loss of Sarah. It was easier to talk with the other parents than to speak with our friends and family about it. There were only one or two of my friends outside the group to whom I spoke about what I was experiencing. Most people didn't want to talk about it and thought since I was pregnant again, I was moving on. I don't blame any of them since it is a natural reaction to avoid speaking of bad things.

The first time I re-entered the nursery after losing Sarah was about two weeks prior to my due date, November 4th. It was extremely difficult and I have to thank one of my friends for putting it in perspective for me. She asked me if the nursery was just for our first baby or if it was where all of our children would spend their first years. I thought about it and realized it would be for all of our children.

We left everything as it was since we originally decorated it in a neutral pattern. There were several things removed and packed away in Sarah's keepsake box, such as the Baby's First Christmas outfit my sister bought, my baby sweater my Grandma made for me and gave to me at my shower, the keepsake christening hat/hankie made by one of my closest friends and a few other items.

As we approached November 4th, thirty seven weeks, I got really crazy. The anxiety of waiting to see if this baby was also going to die was way too much for me. I scheduled an amniocentesis to ensure proper lung development, for November 3rd. We arrived at the hospital at seven thirty A.M. and the amniocentesis was completed quickly. I was hoping my water would just break from the amniocentesis and I would stay in the hospital and start labor. That didn't happen. They sent me home to wait for the results, which I assumed I would receive in a couple of hours.

By mid-afternoon I was really starting to panic for two reasons; I hadn't heard anything yet and I wasn't feeling the baby move too much. We went to the doctor's office and he put me on the baby monitor for about an hour and all was fine.

We waited and waited for the results. By seven thirty P.M., I was frantic. We finally received the results at nine P.M. and we were ready to go. My doctor instructed me to go to the hospital in the morning. We arrived again at seven thirty A.M. I went into this delivery thinking it would be fast because this was our second child and I was already three to four centimeters dilated for the past week or so. I was started on an internal cervix softener. After seven hours there was no change.

I really wanted to have this baby on the 4th since Sarah was born on the 5th and at the rate things were going, it looked like we would end up having him on the 5th. Time went by and I was really starting to have some pain and requested an epidural.

Several hours later, still nothing was happening and at seven thirty P.M., they started me on Pitocin to bring on uterine contractions. The Pitocin was cranked all the way up and the doctor broke my water. Finally things were starting to progress.

Around one A.M. on the 5th, my epidural wasn't working well, so they administered a boost and it was too much and I started to lose feeling from my waist up. This also made me violently ill and I proceeded to vomit for the next hour or so. I was seven centimeters dilated and just wanted the baby out.

I fell asleep for a bit and when I woke up, I felt like I needed to push. It was three fifteen A.M. I asked my doctor how long he thought I would have to push according to where the baby was and he said about an hour. That wasn't going to happen. I started pushing and thirty seven minutes later Jack Peter was born weighing eight pounds, ten ounces. He was twenty one inches long. I remember John and my sister telling me to open my eyes because he was coming out and my doctor laid him on my stomach and I just fell apart. He wasn't crying and they took him over to the warming bed and there was a team of doctors with him. I remember thinking, *He is dead*. I don't hear anything and all these people are working on him. Then I heard him cry and I didn't think I could cry anymore than I was already, but I was wrong. I was so happy to hear noise.

Jack had fluid in his lungs and they also thought he might have broken his collarbone when he came out. When they finished checking him out, they brought him over to me and I was amazed as to how much he looked like Sarah. The exception was their hair. Sarah had dark curly hair and Jack's was straight. It was amazing to look down and see my baby moving, making noises and crying. With Sarah, we didn't have that and it's unbelievable.

They took him to the NICU and he was there for half a day and checked out fine. The fluid had cleared and his collarbone wasn't broken.

I was glad he was in the NICU since he was receiving one-on-one care. I went down during the specified hours to feed him and he was doing well.

We brought Jack home November 7th, a wonderful event. My sister decorated our house with all "It's a Boy" stuff and had a Mickey Mouse lawn sign with his name. It was a joyous day.

I thought this was great, Jack was here and the terrible worrying was over. Wrong…now it's a whole new set of worries. It took me awhile to be able to put him to bed and not just watch him sleep to make sure he was breathing and moving around. I still wake up and check the video monitor throughout the night.

Jack is now nine months old and doing great. I'm still dealing with the loss of Sarah and still angry about losing her. Every day, when I look at Jack, I'm thankful for the gift of him. He has brought such tremendous joy to our lives. I cannot imagine life without him. I also thank Sarah, because if it weren't for her, Jack wouldn't be here…yet.

PATTY

Losing Hope

Heaven needed another angel so they chose you.
Author Unknown

Another birthday already, what a happy day, what a bittersweet day. Only one cake but there should be two. I look at Helena and thank God she is here and one lone tear rolls down my face as I think of her sister, Hope.

It took Stephen, my husband, and me three years to even get pregnant. Three years of treatment for infertility. When we finally got a positive blood test back I thought it was a dream! The day of our first sonogram, the doctor was looking and looking and I thought something was wrong but it wasn't…it was TWINS! The tears, this was great, not one but two; something finally went our way.

I was due in May. I felt great, I was the happiest I had been in years! When I started to spot in January I knew something was wrong. I went for a sonogram and after two techs scanned me, I demanded to know what was going on. One of them blurted out, "It looks like an incompetent cervix." In other words, my body wasn't able to hold the babies, my cervix started to thin out already but it was way too early. I was only twenty four weeks! I had an emergency cerclage and began ninety percent bed-rest until thirty six weeks.

It all happened so fast; all I remember was crying and praying all would go well. And everything did: the stitch held, the babies were getting bigger, I was getting steroid shots for their lungs, just in case I went early.

At thirty five weeks I awoke with a nagging backache and couldn't get rid of it so off to the hospital we went again. I was hooked up to a fetal monitor and my doctor found I was in labor with the cerclage still in place, which isn't a good thing. So I lay there thinking nothing was going right for us. They removed the cerclage, which hurt because I was two centimeters dilated and pulling against the stitch.

I was admitted to wait and see if they could hold off labor. Since I was so far along they wouldn't give me any drugs to delay delivery. They would only keep me on one hundred percent bed-rest until I hit thirty six weeks. The less I was moving the better.

Here I was again. After two days the doctors decided I could get up and walk around and use the bathroom. Thank you, God.

On the last night in the hospital I got out of bed to go to the bathroom and as I stood I got a big gush of fluid. My mom called the nurse. The L&D team came running, I was hooked up to the fetal monitor, and they did an internal exam, taking swabs and telling me they would be right back.

I found out I only peed on myself. How embarrassing! After all of the excitement I got ready to go home the next day.

As I left the hospital it was beautiful out. Spring was here. I was off of bed rest and that felt good. I got permission from my doctor to go to Easter dinner with my family and things couldn't be better.

The babies were doing great. They were moving all the time; you could see movement through my shirt that barely fit me because I was HUGE. I loved every minute of it. We were still trying to pick out baby names. We began to feel we were out of the woods.

Easter was a great day. The whole family tried to guess what we were having, and were helping us pick names.

As we left my dad's house all I could think of was next year we would have two little kids to do an egg hunt with and we would have a family of our own.

At home, I felt a wet dribble and then a full gush as I ran for the shower. I called the OB thinking, *Please let this be my water and not pee.*

My OB told me to put on a pad and call him in an hour. So one hour and four pads later he was sure my membranes had ruptured. He told me to go to labor and delivery and be ready to become parents!

We waited to call everyone; we wanted to make sure I was admitted.

Labor progressed. I told Stephen I couldn't do this and maybe we should wait a day or two. I asked for an epidural. The anesthesiologist gave me so much medicine I slept through my whole labor. At six A.M. I was wheeled to an operating room to deliver, just in case I needed a C-section (we knew twin number two was breech).

Now in the operating room there were so many people I lost count: two neonatal teams, one for each baby, and my doctor and the head of OB/Gyn there to deliver.

By the time I was prepped and everyone was there and ready to go I pushed four times. They told us the baby had a full head of hair and it was a girl! A girl! I wouldn't tell anyone but I wanted a girl so badly.

We were asked her name: Helena, Helena Ann. She was handed off to the neonatologists to work on because she was considered a preemie. Now to deliver my second baby.

After a quick sonogram and the doctors trying to turn the next baby, I was told to start pushing, they were going to deliver the baby breech. I was told this baby was only four to five pounds and since Helena was six pounds they thought there would be no problem.

After an hour of pushing and begging for a C-section we heard my doctor say, "Another girl." Another girl, how could one mom be so lucky? My doctor said good-bye, he'd see me later…he had another delivery.

But the room was silent, no crying. Why no crying? All I heard was doctors yelling, the head neonatologist saying, "Give me a round of Epi, blood gases stat." Stephen was gone; they kicked him out of the room. He got in the doctors' way so they made him stand outside until I begged for him. My doctor reappeared, telling me to give the doctors some time. Still no crying. Then my doctor came over and told me the words we NEVER thought we would hear, "Sorry, Patty, she didn't make it, she passed away."

I looked at him in total shock and asked if I would have to bury her. What a dumb question, but it was the first thing that came into my head. As

I asked this question they brought me my little girl, head full of hair. She had ten fingers and ten toes. They asked me for a name. *Now I have to name her, too?* I told them I don't have one, and I would name her later.

We called my family and told them we delivered. My mom and others arrived. She was so happy. But how do you tell your mom one of her grandchildren just died? This wasn't like a broken vase you could hide. I don't remember her reaction to my saying, "Mom, the second twin died and it was a girl."

The nurses asked me if I wanted to see my baby again. In minutes I was holding her. So beautiful! She looked like she was sleeping. She was dressed in a white dress with yellow trim, a pink and white blanket and matching hat and booties. As I held her, the nurse took a Polaroid. This would be the only picture of me holding her I would ever have.

We passed her around the room and everyone got a chance to hold her, except Stephen. He didn't want to. But after much persuasion he held her, something he was happy he did.

As the nurses took away the baby they brought me Helena, and my doctor walked in. He looked at Helena and he smiled but also he had a sad look in his eyes. Besides being my OB he was also my infertility doctor. He knew how much we wanted the girls. He came to me with a paper in his hand and asked me to have an autopsy performed. I started to freak. But he went on to explain they wanted to know what happened and if maybe she had a birth defect, so I agreed and signed the papers.

My dad walked in. I looked at him and he at me and he began to cry, something I never saw before.

He wheeled me up to my room. I found a stack of papers on my nightstand, all about loss and funerals, plots, burials. I could not believe this was happening. I pinched myself. At least I had a private room. I found out they did this so I could have my privacy to make my arrangements.

Before I could do anything I waited for Stephen. He had gone home to call his parents, who live in Georgia. By the time he got back I was settled and had seen a social worker.

We were happy for the girl we had and sad for the one we lost.

Through a recommendation we found a funeral director, Phil, who was a godsend. He did everything for us.

Now we had to name our angel. Stephen left it up to me; whatever I wanted was fine. The next morning I gave her the name Hope. Hope, what we always had: we hoped we would get pregnant; we hoped the babies would be healthy, so the name seemed to fit.

We had Helena and Hope on Monday, April 5th and were planning to leave on Wednesday and bury Hope on Saturday. Things went pretty well until we got ready to leave. The nurses told me Helena had to stay; she was jaundiced and had to be under the lights. All I could think was I was supposed to leave the hospital with two babies, now I was leaving with nothing.

My OB was great. He made it possible for me to stay almost until Helena was ready to go home. For now everything was all right or as all right as it could be. Every morning my OB sat with me. I was always the last person on his rounds. We would sit and talk. He even fed Helena.

By Friday everything was in place for the funeral, but Helena still had to be under the lights. I left the hospital without her. Looking back it was the best thing I could have done.

At home I took a shower and went to the store to return the second car seat and take all of the doubles off my registry. That was when I found out how cruel people were going to be.

The customer service woman at the store was head of the twins' club and started to grill me on my doctor and what he did wrong on my labor and many other things. By the time she was done I wanted to punch her in her face! I left the store feeling worse.

At home again, I shut off the phone and took a nap. After dinner, Stephen and I wanted to see Helena, so we called the nursery and they told us to come over, they had a surprise for us. When we got there Helena was out of the lights and in the regular nursery. We fed her and changed her but she still had to stay.

Saturday was a beautiful day. We were going to bury our baby. We left home to meet Phil at the cemetery. As we were waiting we saw a hearse pull up and it looked like it was empty but it wasn't, it was Phil with our little angel. Her casket was so small, all I wanted was to hold her again, but I knew I couldn't. I wanted to see her one last time but Phil talked me out of having a wake or even opening the casket. He wanted me to have a good memory of her.

As we talked he pulled an envelope from his jacket, in it was a picture of Hope all dressed in the white and pink dress my friends bought for her. He said she looked so beautiful he had to do that for me.

We went to the grave. The priest arrived and so did my whole family. The priest gave a beautiful service and each family member laid a long-stemmed pink rose on her casket. Before we knew it, it was over. It was all so final.

After the funeral we called the hospital, and they told us they had a surprise. Helena's bilirubin numbers were down and we could take her home. What a bittersweet day, we buried one daughter and got to take the other one home.

Going home proved a little too much for us to handle so we went to my dad's house. At least when the phone rang it was not for us. It wasn't people to say how sorry they were or could they do anything. At this point the only thing they could do was

A) bring back my daughter or

B) leave me alone.

Since no one could do A, than choice B it was.

Things went pretty well as long as I was busy, but if I had too much time to think, that was the end of me. I spent a lot of time at the cemetery. I would sit on the grass and feed Helena, talk to Hope, and cry. The biggest shock was the day her plaque came in, it was so strange to see our last name on a plaque and know it was our daughter. That crying jag lasted for about two days.

For Helena I think visiting there was good. No matter when we went she would always wake up and start to babble like she knew where she was. Even to this day Helena still knows which plaque is Hope's though we only go on the holidays now.

I went back to work the first week in August. It was hard.

Did I want to answer all the questions: *Did you sue your doctor? Why did she die?* The autopsy came back with no cause: no knot in the cord, no placental abruption, everything looked good. The cause: lack of oxygen, and what caused that we will never know.

My co-workers tried to keep the questions from me. I always got one or two of them but I tried to be nice. My favorite was the customer who kept asking me about the twins and I kept saying Helena is doing fine and there was only one and she kept insisting there were two so I told her point blank, the other baby had died. That was the last time I ever saw her.

I have to say as time goes by things do get a little easier. Will I ever forget my angel named Hope? No, NEVER. But as they say out of something bad comes something good. I've made some awesome friends, found out who my true friends are, learned I'm strong and I have a great family which turned out to be my best support system. Always remember one thing: if a person doesn't support you or makes you feel bad about grieving don't talk or be around that person, you have to do what's good for you.

Having Emma

Life is not measured by the number of breaths that we take,
but by the moments that take your breath away.
Author Unknown

It was the summer of 2002. I only did fertility treatments in the spring and summer because I can't imagine being pregnant in the summer. I hate the heat. We tried to get pregnant the summer before but it didn't work and when I was told to stop mid-cycle I almost had a break down.

We didn't want to do in-vitro. This cycle went well, we had eggs, everything looked good. Now was the waiting game: would I get a period or not?

When my period was three days late, I made an appointment for a blood draw. The results take a day. It was the longest twenty four hours of my life. I finally got the call I was waiting for: positive, but I was told the [HCG] numbers weren't high enough. I shouldn't tell anyone because they weren't too sure if I'd miscarry.

I had to go back in forty eight hours for my next blood test. My numbers went up but not enough. So it was another forty eight hours. This went on for a week and a half. Finally we got a definite yes!! Oh, my God. We're pregnant again. *Would everything go OK? Was I setting myself up again?* I can't go through losing another child.

At six weeks I went for my first of many sonograms. There it was, a tiny flutter on the screen. The tears just rolled down my face. After all of the blood-work there it was, a little life. I was given my due date: May 12th. My pregnancies would mirror each other: I was due May 5th, the first time. I tried not to think of this and tried to be happy and not worry.

Time to tell the family. Everyone was happy and just as scared as I was.

After the first sonogram the morning sickness kicked in, a sign of a healthy pregnancy. So far, so good. The doctor planned a cerclage for around twelve weeks. Once that was in place I would feel better. Everything was going smoothly until the first shoe dropped.

As I was cooking dinner one night I felt a big gush. I ran to the bathroom to find blood all over my underwear. Oh no! This could not be happening. Thank God my mom was over, she watched Helena while Stephen and I went to the doctor. Another sonogram and everything looked fine. The baby had a good heartbeat and was spinning. A big sigh of relief.

Now here was the kicker: bed-rest for the next week.

We got to twelve weeks with no more problems. We went to have the cerclage and I was running a fever. The obstetrician and anesthesiologist decided to proceed. All went well and I spent the next eight hours in recovery because I couldn't feel my feet. When I could finally wiggle my toes I was sent home.

All I had to do was stay sane through the next six months. I joined a SPALS group, which helped a lot. One week I went to SPALS, the next week a sonogram and a doctor's appointment, and then back to SPALS again. That way I was always in touch with someone. I also was allowed to hear the baby's heartbeat whenever I needed; all I had to do was call. I only did once or twice. Going for the sonograms made me feel even better. They even did a cord Doppler to make sure the blood was flowing right. I had so many sonograms I filled a picture book with them.

Everything went pretty well until I hit thirty weeks. I started to have contractions and was put on modified bed-rest. Down the stairs once a day, up the stairs once a day. Kind of hard since we live on the second floor.

Close to the end of my pregnancy my anxiety rose. I found myself shaking my belly or drinking orange juice to make the baby move. I always made sure I wore something red to ward off the evil eye. I would try anything. The closer I got to the end the less I talked about the baby. I was afraid to get attached, I was afraid I would lose this baby, too.

All hell broke loose at thirty five and a half weeks. My blood pressure kept going up. Every time I went to the doctor I ended up in the hospital for observation. Now instead of once a week, I was seeing the doctor every other day and every other day I wound up in the hospital. They wouldn't induce me because my pressure would drop after an hour, and all the blood-work came back fine, so, home I would go.

After awhile we stopped running to the hospital right away because I was always sent home. We even made a deal with the doctor that I would go after Stephen got home so I didn't have to leave Helena somewhere. Helena even got tired of this; she wanted to know if this baby would ever come out.

With all of this, the stitch was finally removed on the 15th of April. It didn't hurt this time, one, two, three and it was done. All we had to do was sit and wait and run back and forth to the hospital. I was there so much I was on a first name basis with all the nurses. We finally got so tired of going back and forth; we talked to the doctor about being induced. The catch was I had to have a lung maturity amniocentesis before the hospital would let my doctor induce. An amniocentesis was one thing I never wanted to have. You hear so many things about amniocentesis that go wrong but I wanted this baby out and I wanted it to be OK. I felt the longer I was pregnant the more of a chance something would go wrong.

We went for the amniocentesis on Tuesday, induction would be the next day. This baby has to be ready because I'm ready, so why not? I got the call from the doctor and it was a no-go. I started climbing the walls, crying to the doctor, pleading and begging to be delivered. Looking back this wasn't a sane thing I was doing, all I wanted was a healthy baby and I was begging a doctor to deliver me when a test says the lungs weren't ready. Not smart.

A few days later, in the early morning I got up to find my bed wet. I was bleeding and in labor. The doctor told me to come to the hospital. Again since my mom was there, thank God, we left Helena sleeping and off we went.

My contractions were five minutes apart and I told Stephen to blow all the lights, hey, it was three in the morning, no one is around.

I was three centimeters dilated and was admitted. Getting to the delivery room wasn't fun, I could barely walk.

With the fetal monitor on I could hear the baby's heartbeat. This made me feel a little better. An epidural brought some relief. At ten centimeters it was time to push. I tried but I was so numb I couldn't feel a thing. We waited for the epidural to wear off. Forty five minutes later I began to have feeling. From there on in everything was a blur.

The nurses set up a pushing bar then took it down, the baby was coming faster then they thought. Then my biggest fear happened: I heard the baby's heartbeat drop. I stopped pushing and became hysterical and asked for a C-section. My doctor reassured me everything was fine and told me to give another push because the baby was crowning.

With every push my doctor was getting just as excited as I was. He knew after this I wasn't having any more kids so he was off the hook. All I heard was everyone saying, "Push, Pat, give a big push," and then it happened. A cry, no silence, a great big cry. This was the best sound I had ever heard.

This baby was crying, my baby was alive.

The next thing I heard was, "It's a girl." A girl! I was sure it was a boy. A name. Emma, Emma Rose. Then as Stephen cut the cord I looked at her and she looked just like Hope. Full circle, everything became full circle.

The tears of happiness, sadness, and relief just took over. The doctors checked Emma over and she was given a clean bill of health, six pounds, twelve ounces, nineteen inches. Her birthday, April 26, 2003.

Then something important happened. My fear was gone and I felt happy. I got to call my friends and family and tell them good news. First mom and Helena. Helena all along told me I was having a girl but then to Helena everyone has a girl. Then my dad and his wife, then my friends at work. I saved the best for last: my SPALS group. They were truly happy for me but I was also hoping for them that things could have a happy ending.

The first time I saw Helena and Emma together it gave me a feeling of loss. It should have been two from the start, but it's also a happy feeling to see my girls together. Helena thinks Emma is a doll. Before Emma's arrival we took Helena to sibling class so she knew how to feed and change her, a little mom.

I waited to feed Emma when I knew Helena was coming. What a smile, she had a new little sister. For me it took a while to bond with Emma. I was always afraid something would happen and I would only have one again. For Stephen it was love at first sight. Right after she was born she had him all wrapped up. He would sit and rub her forehead and she would coo for him.

A year has passed since my day in the labor and delivery ward, and I find we take too much for granted. The first step, the first smile, so we sit back and try to enjoy what we have and realize we are lucky we finally have our two girls. Not the way we had planned, but we have them.

CINDY

The Tragic Timeline

And the world thought I had it all but I was waiting for you.
"A New Day" written by Aldo Nova and Stephan Moccio

Brian and I were living the life we always dreamed of together. We married after dating twelve years. We were lucky enough to get pregnant three years later, which was when we purchased our first home.

Our first son was born in July 1998. What a thrill. He was close to three weeks late and nine hours after being induced, Kyle graced us with all of his ten pounds, two ounces. He was gorgeous! We couldn't take our eyes off him. We were amazed the two of us created such a miracle.

I'd developed a fever during the end of my delivery so Kyle was taken to the NICU. They wanted to run some tests to be sure he was healthy. We were devastated that our first child was in intensive care. We didn't have him in the room with us all day as we had hoped. We weren't able to have family and friends walk to the nursery and view our beautiful son. We had to leave the hospital without our child. That was more than I thought I would ever be able to handle.

In the end, Brian and I were able to take Kyle home after all his tests came back negative. What got us through those days was looking at our child in the NICU compared to some of the other babies there. We knew in our hearts Kyle was fine and this was all a precaution. Looking back now, I remember how badly Brian and I felt for the parents of the critical babies who would visit their children day after day. I remember thanking God that we weren't in one of their situations. Little did we know then what was in the cards for our future.

After fourteen months of Kyle-heaven, we were pregnant again. The thrills just kept on coming.

I didn't want to know the sex of my first child, but through a sonogram I found out I was having another boy. Brian loves the element of surprise and never wants to know the sex until the birth. I told him I knew the sex of the baby but made him a promise I wouldn't tell a single person so he would be the second to know. I kept my promise and didn't tell a soul.

July 10, 2000, our millennium baby, Jonathan, was born, weighing eight pounds, nine ounces. I was induced one week after my due date. He came fast. The delivery was incredible this time around. My favorite doctor delivered Jonathan and everything was perfect.

Your first is your first and there's always something special about that. The time you spend with your first is always the most precious because you're experiencing everything for the first time together.

Kyle was a screaming baby but a perfect toddler. To this day, he is such a good boy and a treasure. Jonathan was such a good baby. I always referred to him as my angel baby. I bonded with Jonathan immediately. I think it probably had something to do with the fact he was our second and we weren't as uptight. I remember telling my mother every day how in love I was with Jonathan. He was the perfect baby and a terrible toddler. He gave us a run for our money and continues to do so to this day. He's a real sweetie pie.

June 2001 is when our life would change dramatically. Life in our family seemed to be perfect. We were a family of four with a pooch, in the midst of reconstructing the home we loved. It's still a mystery, with all that was going on and two full-time working parents, how we managed to conceive our third child. We were ecstatic! I had an ovary removed after Jonathan was born so the fact we got pregnant with such little effort came as a bit of a surprise to us. This was the most perfect pregnancy of the three. All tests came back normal, no amnio needed. We just kept plugging along waiting for April 25, 2002.

I felt great. At our twenty week sonogram, Brian and I had our typical talk before the appointment regarding whether we should find out the sex. As always, Brian wanted to wait. I'm sure it's no surprise to say I was itching for my little girl. I adore my boys and am thrilled I had them exactly the way I did. They are such a joy to watch grow up together, even when they're killing each other.

This is going to sound terrible to some who read this; others will know exactly how I felt. Part of me wanted to wait to find out the sex because I thought if I found out I was having another boy, I would be disappointed for the rest of the pregnancy. Once you deliver the child and see it, the gender is a complete non-issue. You immediately fall in love, no matter what.

Before entering the sonogram room, I was set on not finding out the sex. We would wait until the delivery. My gut was telling me I was having another boy. When the sonogram tech asked if I wanted to know the sex, I immediately said YES. It was as if something took possession of my tongue. She asked me what I thought I was having and I said another boy. When she told me I was having a little girl, my heart dropped. I wanted to jump off the table and do a jig. I was so excited. Now I was thinking, *How will I ever be able to keep this excitement to myself?*

I wasn't able to keep my promise to Brian. I was bursting with excitement and had to share. Who's the first person you'd share it with? Your own mother, of course! I'm not sure who was more excited, she or I. I also shared the news with Margaret, our sitter, the second mother to my boys. She takes care of and loves our children as if they were her own. She, too, was thrilled.

I contemplated redoing our nursery and incorporating some more feminine colors into it. I didn't want to give the surprise away so I decided to leave it as it was. I purchased a few pieces of clothing for her, which I hid very well. Our life continued to be chaotic, but we were so happy.

March 25, 2002, our dog Cody developed an immune deficiency disease. He was shipped back and forth daily to different vet hospitals so he would have care twenty four hours a day. He was on death's door. The medication wasn't kicking in and Cody was severely ill.

Brian asked me to make a decision as to what we should do. Cody was really my first boy and I was in my eighth month and my hormones were going nuts. I couldn't make the decision to put my dog to sleep—no way. Within the next week or so, Cody pulled through and continues to live a happy dog life. He bounced back to the dog he was and continues to entertain our family.

I was having terrible stomach pains three weeks before my actual due date. It was Easter Sunday and I was expecting a house full of company. The pain continued to worsen. Since I had to be induced with my other two children, I wasn't really sure what it felt like to be in natural labor. These pains were so bad and coming on stronger and quicker, I thought for sure I was in labor. Off we went to the hospital. Our company came to our home as planned.

It turned out I had a stomach virus and was puking after a couple of hours. I was sent home and spent the entire day in bed. I can't tell you how many times I think back to this day wishing I was in labor.

Somewhere in early April, I happened to catch an episode of "A Baby Story." During the episode, one mom was in labor, the baby was in distress and they had to perform a C-section. It turns out the cord was around the baby's neck. They were able to save the child and you are left to think they go on to live happily ever after. The visions from this show remained in my head. I remember thinking, *Thank God this happened in the hospital or the baby would have been lost.*

The bad thoughts were heavy on my mind toward the end of this perfect pregnancy. I never experienced anything like it before. I remember walking down my hallway, looking into the nursery and saying to myself, *What would I do if I weren't able to bring this baby home? What would we do with everything?* Never a thought with my other pregnancies.

April 19th, I had a regular doctor appointment. Everything was perfect. I asked what their intentions were with this child and could they induce me. My doctor told me they couldn't before my due date without good reason. Nothing was going on with my cervix so I had to wait it out.

April 24th Brian was working late so I took my kids to Friendly's for dinner. My niece Megan joined us. Thank God she was there because I was in space a bit. I remember sitting in a booth by the window and rubbing my stomach the entire time. With the third pregnancy, you definitely take the movement factor for granted, especially when your life is so busy. You aren't as in tune to every movement as you are in the first pregnancy.

This was the first time I thought the movement might have slowed down a lot. I remember thinking the baby has less room to move and they always move less toward the end. I didn't do a good job convincing myself. I was awake for most of the night rubbing and poking. I was waiting for a response from my baby. At four A.M., I felt something. Not sure what it was, but I now realize it wasn't my baby moving. But that little movement was what relaxed me enough to finally fall asleep.

I was planning on calling the doctor in the morning to go in for a checkup. My normal appointments were on Saturday, but I thought it would be best for me to go in the next day.

I woke up feeling cramps. As the morning progressed, I felt even more of them. Not sure exactly what could be going on, I decided to go on with my regular routine. I sent Kyle to pre-school and Jonathan to the sitter and decided to work from home, finalizing things before my maternity leave. I was scheduled for one P.M. As the day went on and I continued feeling more and more pain, my Aunt Chris told me I better get my butt to the hospital. If this child was going to come as fast as Jonathan, I better get moving.

I called Brian and told him to come home and take me to the hospital. For some reason, he wanted me to go to the doctor and call him from there to let him know what to do. He told me he had some things to wrap up at work knowing he might be out for the next few days. I was so annoyed and angered with his response and I said something I regret to this day. I told him if anything happened to the baby, or me, it would be his fault. It's not even like me to say something like that.

I packed up the car with my hospital bag, bags for the kids and the dog. I was planning to be gone for a few days. My husband didn't have a bag prepared for him. After he just annoyed me I wasn't about to put one together for him. The hospital I was delivering at was nearly an hour from my home. I picked up the kids, then decided to give my mom a call to meet me at the doctor's office so she could sit with the kids while I went in for the exam. That was the best decision I made.

At one P.M. on April 25th time stood still. I went into the exam room and didn't say anything about the lack of movement, as I was so anxious to hear my baby's heartbeat. That never happened. There was no heartbeat with the Doppler so my doctor asked me to come with him to a room where there was a sonogram machine. Now my heart was beating out of my chest. All I remember is hearing the words, "I'm sorry." My reaction was slightly delayed. I was in total shock. I asked him to have someone get my mom. Once I saw her and told her my baby died, I totally lost it. I guess saying the words myself made it real. I kept hearing, "I'm so sorry."

I needed to call Brian. I wasn't sure how to do that knowing he was at work thinking the next call he got from me was to meet him at the hospital to deliver our child. I couldn't even bring myself to make the call.

My mom tried to do it and she fell silent. She handed the phone to the doctor who explained what happened. I think some nurses were in the waiting room with my children but I wasn't even thinking of them.

I was in a fog. The only word I could use to describe it is surreal—like it was a nightmare from which I was supposed to awaken. When my brother got there he was hugging me so tightly. I remember saying to him, "Vin, this was my little girl." He lost it with me. Remember, no one knew we were having a girl.

When Brian got to the doctor's office, I held him and couldn't let go. I said the same thing, "Brian, this was our little girl." He was numb from the point he got the phone call. He had no idea what to do. The two of us together were pathetic.

Now the four of us were in the office with the doctor and we had to start making decisions. I had to deliver this baby naturally. I had a choice to either do it this day or the next. I had to decide, Brian was just numb. I have no idea where my strength was coming from, but I needed to get this over with as soon as possible. I couldn't bear the thought of sleeping through the night knowing my dead baby was inside and I did nothing to stop it from happening. I know now there isn't anything I could have done, but guilt is the first thing you feel.

We told our doctor we had to get the kids settled at my mom's and then we'd meet one of the other doctors from the practice at the hospital. We went to Brian's mother's home to tell her what happened. She was so upset for us but when we left I almost felt she was telling us maybe there's been some type of mistake. I'm not sure if she was trying to make us feel better or herself.

We must have taken a long time to get to the hospital because my doctor was there, waiting for us to arrive.

The nurses were incredible. They did everything as quickly as they could for me.

Thank God, the process itself went fast. I was hooked up to the Pitocin, and told I could have my epidural as soon as I wanted it. Within an hour, I was given my drugs.

Quickly I was at ten centimeters and things were starting to happen. I remember feeling like my bottom was on fire; my baby's head was coming and my doctor wasn't even in the room. The nurses had to coach me through the delivery and at the last second, Dr. X appeared out of breath. He wasn't expecting me to go so quickly. I remember hoping and praying with all I had left maybe there was some mistake and my baby would come out crying. That never happened. There was silence—what a horrible sound.

Seeing my husband's face through this all was something I'll never forget. He was so worried about me and I was so worried about what he was going to see. No one prepares you for what's to come next. I never thought I was going to be able to see my baby. I thought it would be too much. I even told Brian to look at me and not look at what was going on, but how could you not look? Based on what Brian, the nurses, and the doctor said, we lost our baby because the umbilical cord was wrapped around her neck. The same cord that kept her alive for nine months inside of me killed our baby girl.

When asked if we wanted an autopsy performed, we immediately said no. We were comfortable with the information we were given. The doctor told me, based on the way she looked, this had happened pretty recently. If only I'd insisted they induce me at my last appointment, I could have been home already with my baby.

We had to decide when and if we wanted to see our baby. We knew we had to have our time with her. The nurses dressed her in a dress with a pink knit hat and a pink blanket and brought her into us. She was the most beautiful thing we had ever seen. Her face was a little bruised, but she looked perfect to us and at peace. I wish I had thought to bring the outfit I bought for her. I hated the dress they had her in. I wanted to dress her up and make her look even prettier. Brian and I unwrapped her blankets and checked out every inch of her little precious body. I couldn't stop hugging and kissing her. She looked just like Jonathan, which was a little spooky. She had red hair just like both our dads did as children.

The time we spent with our daughter was so precious. As sad as it was, it was so special and I'm so glad we handled it the way we did. My husband and I cried for what seemed like forever with her in our arms. We couldn't believe we were experiencing this. *Why were we the ones chosen to take this path? Why did God take the little girl I always dreamed of away from me? Why? Why? Why?* She would have completed our almost perfect life. From this moment on, it would never feel perfect again.

Bereavement counselors, social workers, nurses, and doctors visited us. It was all so overwhelming. I remained surprisingly strong through this whole ordeal. We had to choose her name now. We were planning on naming her Victoria after my grandmother. I was so excited knowing the dream I had since I was a little girl was going to come true. She would be Tori for short. Since we didn't know if we would have another girl or if maybe my sister would have a little girl she'd like to name Victoria, we decided her first name would be Angel and her middle Victoria. Angel Victoria Canny, stillborn on April 25, 2002 just before ten P.M.

I don't think I stopped crying the entire night. Moments of strength were few and far between. Brian was as bad. He stayed in the room with me through the night. The nurses did all they knew how to make us as comfortable as possible.

My mom was with my boys. I think I saw every man I know cry for us through this ordeal. It was the saddest thing ever. Part of me was trying to be strong for everyone. It was very strange. Maybe it didn't totally hit me yet. I kept telling everyone I was OK. I was so far from OK I didn't even realize it. Three of our nieces also came to visit. One of them, Erin, was to be Angel Victoria's godmother. This was going to be her first godchild. I was terribly sad for her, too.

A priest came to see us and the nurses performed some type of blessing. Our child wasn't even worth baptizing. We weren't happy about this at all.

Somehow, Brian and I made it through the worst night of our lives. We had to say goodbye to our daughter. I wanted to keep her forever; I didn't want her to go down to a morgue all by herself in some drawer. She was just a baby who needed her parents and whose parents so desperately needed her.

The next morning we couldn't get out of the hospital fast enough. Brian was so touched by the nurses; he couldn't even get the words out to thank them for all they had done. How devastating it was to leave the hospital without our baby. This time we weren't coming back in a couple of days to get her. I felt as if a bus hit me. The pain in my heart was like someone was stabbing me.

We went to my mother-in-law's house to make some more absurd decisions. We didn't go to my mom's because we weren't ready to see our boys just yet. We asked the family priest to come by and help us with the funeral arrangements. We had no idea what we were supposed to do. This was the priest who baptized my husband and me, married us, baptized our boys, and would now help us bury our little girl.

Brian's family is as close to me as my own. He is one of eight children and every member of both families was there for us through this tragedy. His sister Ellen and his mom were waiting for us with lunch. Brian got right on the phone and started making the arrangements with the funeral parlor. He took care of everything. I'm usually who plans and coordinates everything but Brian just took over. I was so proud of the way he did that. I think he had to do it for himself for some reason. I know he was also trying to alleviate the burden on me.

We were ready to see our boys. In fact, we desperately needed them. We decided we weren't going to tell them anything just yet. Kyle was four and Jonathan, two, so we knew we could buy some time. My sister and my mom brought our boys to us.

I was so happy to see those boys. I remember Jonathan would touch my belly every single day, without saying or asking anything, now he just stopped. I knew this child sensed something. I saw Brian with Kyle in his arms. He wouldn't let him go. When I saw my husband's face, he was in tears. It broke my already-broken heart. He was in worse shape than I was for the first couple of days. We have always been a very close and bonded couple, but our bond was strengthening by the minute. Tragedy like this can tear families apart. I did have the fear this could happen. I spoke about it with Brian. We weren't going to allow ourselves to be broken.

I was physically and emotionally drained. At my mom's later that day, she found me crying on her bed. I thought I was never going to sleep again. It was a terrible feeling. I didn't want any medication. I wanted to work it through on my own.

That night Brian held me and I was able to get some rest. He had to do this often; it was the only way I was able to fall asleep. I thank God for the husband I have. I know I've been blessed to have him as my life partner.

Saturday, April 27th, we should have been coming home from the hospital with our beautiful little girl. Instead, we were at the funeral home making arrangements to bury her. Surreal.

We had to purchase an outfit in which to bury her. We went to a little boutique close to our home that has the most adorable clothes. We found a white outfit with pink flowers on it. When we went to pay for it, the woman asked if we were bringing home a baby. I replied, "You don't even want to know what we're doing with this outfit."

With that, I had to leave the store. I was hysterical again. Brian told this poor woman our story. She felt terrible. She started throwing a blanket, hat, and shoes at no charge. He told her we would be back one day on a happier note. (I did return almost two years later to purchase my son's christening outfit. The woman remembered me, and what Brian said to her that day. She was thrilled I came back on a happier note). Next stop was the florist and the caterer. We were on automatic pilot.

On Monday, Brian dropped our children off with our sitter. We didn't want them exposed to all the sadness. The night before the funeral, we finally got enough courage together to explain what had happened to their sister. We were honest with them but kept in perspective the fact they were so little. They were sad but reacted better than we expected. It worked out fine.

Brian and I went to the funeral home before the Mass we had scheduled at our church. We didn't have a wake. It was way too much for people to handle. We went in alone to see our daughter for the last time. My family waited outside as we requested.

Angel Victoria looked like a little angel. So beautiful in the outfit. I put pictures in her coffin and a teddy bear so she wouldn't be alone. I gave her the cross my mom had given to me when I received my confirmation. I had jewelry for Angel Victoria from my mom and my sister. Standing in front of

Angel's little coffin, all I wanted was to take her with me. It wasn't natural to leave our daughter in a box all alone. She was so tiny and she needed us to take care of her.

I hurt so badly. Brian and I said our last goodbye and started leaving the funeral home. I asked Brian if he thought it would be all right if my mom saw her. Mom wanted to see her but I was afraid of how she would react so I said no. After seeing how beautiful she looked, I couldn't deny the request. Brian agreed.

My mom needed closure for her own grieving process and I had to give that to her. She handled it better than I expected and is forever grateful to us for giving her a moment with her granddaughter.

We requested the car with our daughter be outside the church and that the coffin not be brought in. Just its size would have upset people. We didn't want that nor did we think we could handle it. I knew for sure she was there with us in spirit. I sat in church with my husband squeezing one hand and my brother squeezing the other. My brother, sister-in-law, and my one-year-old niece, Maxine Victoria, sat next to us. I watched my brother cling to his wife and daughter. I was touched by this and thought, *Yes, Vinny, hold on tight and don't ever let her go*. Thank God for my special niece. I treasure her deeply and am lucky to have her close to me for the tough days.

The number of people at the mass was overwhelming. Brian and I were touched with the love and support. We requested that only immediate family and closest friends come to the cemetery. We wanted more of an intimate ceremony. Angel Victoria was being buried with my dad who died thirty years before. He never saw his own children grow up so I wanted to give him one of his grandchildren.

It was quite an emotional thing for us all. Leaving the cemetery was a horror. Some of our loved ones were saying, "She's with your dad now." I still wanted her to be coming home with me where she really belonged.

We had everyone back to our house for lunch. The first thing I wanted to do was get my hands on my boys. Brian was feeling the same exact thing so he went with my brother-in-law to get them. Those two boys will never know how they changed the faces of everyone when they walked in. They got more kisses and hugs than they ever bargained for. Our boys got us through this. They kept our minds diverted. We would look at them and thank God we were blessed with them.

Brian and I joined a bereavement group through Winthrop University Hospital. It went on for six weeks. It was a tremendous help to us. We surrounded ourselves with our family and close friends, which helped as well. We tried to get away from our day-to-day life with some type of trip.

We vacationed a couple of times until our friends told us they could no longer afford to be friends with us; we traveled so much we were making everyone else broke in the process.

It is now two years and seven months since we lost our daughter. I think about her every day. She will always be a part of our family. My heart still aches for our child in heaven. I just want to know she's safe and happy. I don't think I'll ever really know. I can only hope some day I'll join her again.

An Angel in Disguise

A new day has begun.
"A New Day" written by Aldo Nova and Stephan Moccio

I felt I could never go through this kind of loss again. That phase lasted a very short period of time—maybe a day. The next feeling was to get pregnant again right away. I would think, *Am I just thinking I can replace her?* That wasn't possible so I gave myself the time to grieve and heal emotionally before getting pregnant. My own personal timeline was around a year.

After losing my child, I went to get my own body checked out to make sure I worked fine. I had a complete physical and blood tests. I returned to a neurologist for what was thought to be a neurological problem. I've since understood the symptoms I'd felt then and again after losing my child were from anxiety. I had a D&C five months after delivering Angel Victoria because of irregular periods. The doctors suggested waiting six months since I had had a full term pregnancy; my body needed the time to heal.

Brian was ready whenever I was. He left all the choices totally up to me. I knew he wanted another child, but if my decision were no way, he would have accepted it. Nine or ten months after the loss, I decided we wouldn't prevent a pregnancy any longer. I didn't use any ovulation predictors but I dabbled on some websites to try and figure out how to have a girl after two boys and one girl. I was diligently trying to make a girl according to the rules I found on the website.

Brian thought I was nuts but was always willing to play along. I was thirty five, he thirty six, our boys each a year older. Angel Victoria would have been eleven months. We were all ready for another baby, I thought.

March 2003, the stick showed two PINK lines. So did the next five sticks. I took six tests since we couldn't believe we were blessed again. Pure bliss for a few days, then I started feeling guilty about being so excited. I felt I was cheating on my daughter. I felt bad for not being excited for my new baby. It was the start of the biggest emotional roller coaster I ever rode.

I managed to stop feeling guilty right about the same time the fear of God set in, fear that lasted throughout the pregnancy and still continues to linger.

With all pregnancies, you pray to make it past the first trimester. You tell yourself then your mind will be a little more at ease. That doesn't work when you've lost a full term baby. It just makes you realize there really is no safe time until you're holding the baby in your arms.

I knew about the support groups offered at the hospital. I didn't keep in touch with any of the other couples from our loss-support group. I don't think we ever really had the chance to bond with anyone since almost every couple with the exception of Brian and I missed the group each week. All our connections were formed at the SPALS groups.

We were late starters in our gathering. We started when we were five months pregnant. Thank God we did. I only wish we had started when the fourth stick turned pink. Not only did we form incredible friendships with the other couples, it was what kept us on the level. It was also a time where it was good to talk, grieve, and cry for your lost child. These people knew it was all right to be happy and sad at the same time because they were feeling the exact same thing. Although we had incredible support from the wonderful women who ran the groups, there were many times where we would be the ones to offer the therapy needed to each other.

I was so lucky to have a pretty uneventful pregnancy. I thought about switching OB practices only to choose a practice closer to my home. There wasn't anything my OB did that could have changed the outcome for us. I really do love the doctors in the practice and they knew all my history so I decided to stay with them.

My initial visit was at nine weeks. I couldn't wait to hear the baby's heartbeat. My husband and I heard that wonderful sound and some of the happiness we were missing for the past year started to come back.

We waited until after our initial appointment to share the news with family and friends. Of course, tears were everywhere. We told our boys. We weren't sure if we should wait until I was further along because of what had happened before, but we decided to treat this pregnancy as we had treated the last. The boys were thrilled. They would climb into bed with me in the morning and talk to my belly, touch it, and listen to it. They were so much fun. They were a little bit older so they were a little more involved.

I started enjoying things again during the second and part of the third trimester. We decided against the AFP. I was thirty five and knew the levels would probably come back elevated from that factor alone. I also was a candidate for an amniocentesis but didn't have one; deciding ignorance was bliss this time. What I didn't know wouldn't hurt me.

My next stepping-stone was at twenty weeks, my level II sonogram. We decided we weren't going to find out this time the baby's gender—we were just so happy it really didn't matter.

I was in the room alone with the sonogram technician. She asked me if I wanted to know the sex—my mind said NO but the word YES came screaming out of my mouth.

This baby was another boy. At first, my heart dropped and I will admit I was disappointed for about thirty seconds.

The doctor reported everything was great. From then on, I couldn't stop laughing. The "My Three Sons" theme song kept playing in my head and I just kept laughing. It REALLY didn't matter.

I was blessed with another healthy baby. Brian and the boys came and joined the fun. My smile was from ear to ear so I knew Brian was probably thinking: another girl. I didn't tell him and neither did the doctor.

I wanted so badly to tell him. I finally tortured him into letting me tell him because I thought it was just too good to keep to myself. He was pretty surprised when I told him. I know he will always feel bad we both missed our chance for a girl.

When I told people what we were having, they reacted as if they felt bad for us. I explained it really didn't matter. My sorrow was I could never get our daughter back and I would always feel cheated about not having HER.

My third trimester was probably one of the best. I got used to being pregnant again. My mental state was better—especially with the help of SPALS. I knew I would work up until the end. I didn't want to waste my maternity leave before the baby's arrival. My co-workers are like a second family. My boss was probably the best of the group. Having lost two children himself at five months each time, I knew my situation hit home for him. He tried to be sure I was going to be all right before and after the baby arrived. He and I got our department together for a mini-shower. Cake, gifts, it was so special.

Some people would have possibly steered clear of my situation because of what happened the last time. They didn't. I was impressed and touched.

We decided the baby's name was going to be Jake since I loved it. Brian pretty much let me have my way with anything this time around. His middle name would be Louis, after my grandfather. The boys called my belly Baby Jake. We kept the nursery exactly the same. I never even cleared out all the drawers after losing Angel Victoria. I had my mom over to help me rewash everything. This was emotional for both of us.

The last two weeks before the delivery were the worst. I just kept thinking of what could go wrong. We decided we would deliver at thirty seven weeks after an amnio for lung maturity. Funny thing with this pregnancy, every time I found myself questioning movement, this baby would move. I never felt more connected with any of my other children. It was really amazing. I tortured this poor child for nine months and he responded to every thought and poke. One week before delivery I was a basket case. My husband had to take me to the hospital because I wasn't sure if I felt movement. I wanted this kid out.

Thirty-seven weeks and an amnio was scheduled. Through this entire pregnancy I stayed away from the doctor who delivered my daughter. Guess what? He was the one who performed the amnio and he was fantastic. All went well and we had lung maturity. That same night I was admitted.

Friday, November 7th, I got hooked up to the Pitocin drip at eight A.M. Contractions got stronger and closer together. I got my epidural. The bittersweet feelings returned. I was so anxious about just delivering this baby and getting him in my arms. This was the same hospital. I saw some of the nurses who had taken care of me when I lost Angel Victoria; they remembered us. The room seemed so much brighter to us this time. My mom was supposed to be there for the birth of my daughter, but since it never happened I invited her to see her grandson being born.

This kid came fast and fierce. After only two and a half hours he was ready to come out. I think the staff was even surprised—they rushed to get the room ready.

Just in time, the one and only Dr. X arrived. He had done great by me through this whole ordeal. One and a half pushes later, Baby Jake Louis was born, seven pounds, two ounces. The second before Jake came out, Dr. X told me to raise my head, open my eyes and look.

I have to say for that split second, he scared me. I thought something was wrong again. The next words out of his mouth were, "Cindy, I want you to see your baby being born."

It was the most amazing thing. No doctor has ever done that to me before. I will never forget that moment. Needless to say, now I absolutely love Dr. X! Jake cried, so did his Mommy, Daddy, and Grammy.

It was truly amazing. One of, if not THE, happiest moments of my life. He was perfect.

We couldn't help but think of our previous trip to labor and delivery. This was a much happier outcome, but it was still mixed with a dash of sadness and lots of hurt over the daughter who didn't cry in the silent room.

What got us through the pregnancy? Each other, the never-ending love and support of our families and friends, the SPALS people and meetings twice a month!

If we hadn't lost Angel Victoria, Baby Jake would never have been. I couldn't even picture our lives without Jake. It feels as if one child had to be sacrificed for another—that's the heart-wrenching part. I have to believe she helped him find his way to us. It helped me deal with not having my daughter, but at the same time, made me so very sad. For me, part of Angel Victoria will be in our Jake.

Jake is eleven months old now. He spent the first week back in the hospital with a severe milk protein allergy. That week was torture and started my battle against panic attacks, which is my body's way of saying it couldn't take anymore, I guess.

We made it through. I was medicated with Zoloft and Xanax for a short period of time. It wasn't until now, close to a year later, I decided to speak with a therapist.

What I experienced with Jake in the hospital was a combination of things. One of the main problems was post-traumatic stress disorder. My therapist was stunned I waited so long to seek professional help. I always reached out to close family and friends and thought with their support and my strong will, I would be able to handle this on my own. That was wrong.

After seeing my therapist, the physical symptoms of the anxiety left my body. I'm trying to build up my strength again without medications. I feel I need to be prepared just in case the "other shoe drops." I will always live with the fear in the back of my head, though maybe therapy will make it go away. Only time will tell.

Jake is doing great, so are we all. We enjoy each other thoroughly since we all know how precious life truly is. There will ALWAYS be a hole in our hearts for our Angel Victoria. She will NEVER be forgotten. Jake was a gift that brought some much-needed happiness back in all our lives. He will always be our family treasure.

LYNN V.

My Angel Sara, Who Changed Our Life Forever

In my heart, there will always be a place for you for all my life
And everywhere I am, there you'll be
"There You'll Be" written by Diane Warren

It was the saddest day of my life. May 27, 2001. I had a stillborn baby. This day would change me forever.

I came from a big family, eight children. I lost my mother when I was thirteen. Sara was conceived just the month after my father died in August 2000.

September was my Dad's birthday; he knew I wanted a sister for our daughter, Erin, and son, Richie. Since I have sisters, I wanted Erin to have one, too. I thought my mother and father were finally together and were going to send me a baby girl. I found it out for sure at my twenty week sonogram

It was a good time to change obstetricians since a move to Long Island put my Manhattan OB out of bounds. We chose a group recommended by the hospital in which I would deliver.

In the winter, my son caught Fifth Disease (Parvo Virus B19); I was nervous. My obstetrician did a follow-up blood test to check for antibodies to Fifth Disease and found them.

In April my feet began to swell. I could feel the water swishing around in them. The physicians dismissed it as being from the days of heat we were having. I also went to them for abdominal pain only a couple of weeks before we lost Sara.

Everything was always dismissed. It seemed having two healthy babies already and being only thirty one, it was assumed Sara was healthy, also.

I went for a check up at thirty seven weeks, I told the doctor I wasn't feeling as much movement anymore. He said, "Watch that, and let us know."

Then the dreadful day came.

It was a rainy Memorial Day weekend. Sunday, I felt no movement. We went to the hospital. A physician came in the room to do a sonogram and when he found no heartbeat, he told us she was gone. We were devastated. My husband's immediate reaction was to check the machine. "Check the sonogram, are you sure?" I asked the doctor as he was leaving the room, "What do I tell my children?" He said, "Tell them the truth." It was the worst day of our lives.

Dr. F. from my OB group was on-call. She arrived and encouraged us to let them do an amniocentesis so they can try to see why she died. They tried twice, but I didn't have any fluid left.

She encouraged a natural delivery. Richie, my first born, was a natural birth, but Erin was a C-section. I told her I just wanted a C-section. She said it would be better to have a natural delivery, as I wouldn't be in so much physical pain afterwards because I was going to be in so much emotional pain and I would have to deal with the death of my child.

They began drugs intravenously to bring on contractions. I asked Dr. F to be close by, because I had the drugs with Erin and the contractions came on fast. She left, though, saying she would be back in a couple of hours. I was thrown into labor almost immediately.

By this time, I had HELLP Syndrome (Hemolysis, Elevated Liver Enzyme Levels, Low Platelet Syndrome), a rare form of eclampsia. It became very scary to the doctors around me. I remember my blood pressure shooting up as I began to swell.

I cried and told Rich, "I'm not going to make it." I rocked in my bed yelling. I remember a doctor saying, "She's like a raging animal." Dr. F. returned, frantic, and I kept asking her what was wrong with me.

She said, "I have to stabilize you." They had my head practically hanging upside down, while starting me on blood pressure medicine and magnesium to prevent seizures.

When I was finally stabilized I delivered Sara naturally. I will never forget the silence in the room as I pushed. There was the doctor, a nurse and my very sad husband, who couldn't bear to watch the birth and tried to help me as much as possible.

Sara was so beautiful. I couldn't understand. Perfectly formed but only four pounds, eleven ounces. Her lips were black and she was blue. Her fingernails were blue. I held her for some time and I cried so hard.

We asked for a priest, since we are Catholic, to read her the last rites. But the priest who came was just awful. He didn't speak English well, he appeared under the influence of alcohol, which I smelled on his breath and I couldn't understand a word he said. I was very disappointed.

Two of my sisters and our brother-in-law were in the waiting area. They came in and cried with us. My sister told Rich not to leave me with the baby for a long time; it would only make it more difficult. I didn't know this at the time. The nurse came in and took the baby.

This was the saddest moment of my entire life. I felt horrible. I felt like a terrible mother. *How could I let this happen*? I longed for her so much. I couldn't believe I wouldn't go home with her.

The nurse returned holding a pale green box, with Sara's footprints in it, a Polaroid picture and a small infant shirt and hat she was dressed in after delivery. I didn't want to depart without her. It was so hard to let her go. I wish now I'd kept her with me. I wish I'd changed her, bathed her and dressed her. I wish I kept her in my arms that night.

We were so sad. I wouldn't let them autopsy her. We never quite figured out what happened, but I did have HELLP Syndrome and they attributed placental failure to that. We think it's what caused Sara's death, but we will never be sure.

The magnesium they gave me to prevent seizures made me sick. I had a horrific headache and I cried all night.

The next morning Rich asked to get us out of the room we were in. We had been there more than a day. It was a dark room and we were losing our minds. They finally put us in a very small room by ourselves in the maternity ward. You could hear happy couples outside the room enjoying their families and infants. We lay there silent, alone, depressed. The sadness was so overwhelming. Our lives had changed forever.

A social worker from the hospital came to talk to us and gave us a ton of literature. We read all the sad poems. We cut two out and put them in Sara's green memory box.

This was the day Richie and Erin would come see us and I would have to tell them their baby sister died. They cried a little. They seemed afraid and wanted to leave the hospital. They asked how she died. We had to tell them she stopped breathing. They didn't understand.

When I was released from the hospital the very hardest moment came. I was told I had to be brought to my car by wheelchair instead of walking out. It was hospital policy. So out I went, wheeled through the maternity ward with Sara's green box on my lap, alone. Rich had gone to get the car. It was so hard leaving the hospital without our baby. We had to go home and plan her funeral instead.

I punched the door of our van screaming, "I want to die," as we drove off. I just couldn't bear leaving empty handed, knowing she was in the morgue.

We were in the middle of dormering our house to make room for the baby. Our home was a mess and under construction. Once inside, I collapsed in tears. No one was home. Our kids were in school.

We looked at Sara's picture and went through the things in her box. We went up to the room being built for her. Rich wrote special words to her on the wall, how she will be missed and how we loved her.

When the kids came home we sat with them and read them some of the stories and literature the hospital had provided. They were worried they, too, could stop breathing and we had to explain to them how that wasn't going to happen.

We needed to start the dreaded phone calls. Through our parish we discovered a funeral home that hosts funerals for loss of a child or baby. Later that evening we went there.

As we drove up the sky got very dark. Just as I touched the doorknob to the funeral home, thunder and lightening bolted through the sky. I thought, *She is crying, she is crying for us*. The thought of it was killing me.

I brought an outfit and some little toys for Sara, to be put on her and in her coffin. I forgot to bring a diaper. It almost killed me, I brought toys and clothes and not a diaper for my little girl.

They described the coffin to us and told us the time and arrangements. I asked if I could view her for a moment before we went to the burial. The funeral director said in his exact words, "There is nothing to see." I was appalled at this comment. I said, "What do you mean there is nothing to see? She is beautiful." And he said, "That isn't what I meant, we don't embalm babies. We don't have viewings for them."

At home, I contacted my parish. The priest who called back said he would come to the funeral home and say a prayer for Sara and us over her little white coffin.

The next day, Sara's funeral.

My husband is a police officer. As we walked into the funeral home, the hall was lined with officers, friends and family. We entered the room to her small white coffin with flowers on top of it. I sat there and I wanted so much to open the coffin and hold her. The pain was unbearable.

After the prayer service, we followed her coffin to the cemetery. The police department offered an escort. First past our house, holding up lights and stopping traffic. They led us to her resting place. At the cemetery, Rich read a beautiful poem in her memory.

If tears could build a stairway,
And memories were a lane,
We would walk right up to heaven,
To bring you home again.

No farewell words were spoken,
No time to say goodbye,
You were gone before we knew it,
And only God knows why.
Our hearts still ache with sadness,
And secret tears still flow.
What it meant to lose you,
No one will ever know.
We knew little that day
God was going to call you.
It broke many hearts to lose you,
But you didn't go alone.
For part of us went with you,
The day He called you home.
You left us beautiful memories,
Your love is still our guide,
And though we cannot see you,
You are always by our sides.
-Author Unknown

At the end of the service, we didn't want to leave her. It was so hard. I wanted to grab the coffin and run away with it. I wanted to hold her one more time; I wanted to see her one more time.

Sara is buried in Section twenty three and we visit her all the time, even now, three years later. My parents aren't far from her in Section three. My birthday is 3/23. I think of her all the time. She will never be forgotten, we will always long for her. It is a terrible pain to live with. We wait to meet her some day in heaven.

Rich and I went to a support group a few times and cried with other couples who suffered horrific losses. It was comforting to me to be around people who were going through the same pain. No one understood except those who also had a loss.

We also went to a conference the hospital holds every year for anyone who has lost a baby there. They have a baby memorial garden there, where we plant bulbs every year and Sara has a memorial brick. At the conference, they sing songs like "Amazing Grace" and read poems and end it at the memorial garden where we plant flowers for the spring around the bricks. We bring our children with us. It's a day we dedicate to Sara's memory.

Caitlyn & Anthony, Our Precious Gifts Sent From Heaven, After Sara, Our Angel

With arms wide open
"With Arms Wide Open" written by Scott Stapp

I went to so many doctors for their opinion of what they thought happened to Sara. Should I conceive again? What was HELLP Syndrome and why did I get it? Could I get it again? What were my chances of having a healthy baby? Was there something wrong with me? Was I sick?

I longed so much for a baby, though; I really wanted to try again. Some doctors told me not to chance it, HELLP Syndrome was very serious and could reoccur and since I already had two healthy children, I shouldn't push the envelope, as two of them said. I called the obstetrician who delivered Richie and Erin. He told me to go to Mt. Sinai Hospital Perinatal Group and let them inform me. They were apparently experts in the field. That is where a doctor, who seemed well-informed of HELLP Syndrome, told me I had a thirty percent chance of having it again, but they would watch me closely with blood tests, and sonograms. The doctor thought after studying some blood-work I could definitely try to have a baby again.

That was a relief. I had post-partum high blood pressure for seven months. We were trying to conceive all the while. I hadn't ever needed any help conceiving. I always knew when I was ovulating. I thought I was pregnant in December 2001. I went to my doctor and told her I felt something on my right side and that I had missed my period. She diagnosed an ovarian cyst. I was so upset.

I felt like I wasn't meant to have any more children. Perhaps my parenting was all wrong and I somehow lost Sara because I wasn't a good parent and shouldn't have any more children. I knew then how women who can't conceive must feel and all the thoughts that must go through their minds.

In February 2002, my period was late again, but this time, I went and got two pregnancy tests and took both a couple of days apart. They were both positive. We were thrilled, but worried and frightened all at the same time.

Richie and Erin were so happy, too, but also wondered and asked, "Will this baby stop breathing, too?"

Our doctor confirmed the pregnancy and did an internal sonogram. A hormone count was low and he warned me I might miscarry. My husband and I hoped and prayed, and we didn't.

I searched the Internet for websites on HELLP Syndrome. I found a list for post-HELLP pregnancies. The post-HELLP pregnancy stories were scary. Most were first pregnancies. Most of them all started with some abdominal pain. There was no story exactly like mine. Only two other stories were a third and fourth pregnancy. It was rare what happened to me. Most had good outcomes with their subsequent pregnancies. Some women emailed me and I emailed them. It was a help.

I wondered what our outcome would be.

I went to a high-risk doctor, and he too, was well informed on HELLP Syndrome. He was very positive, yet cautious. I also saw a cardiologist and a blood specialist.

It was a long nine months waiting for Caitlyn's arrival. People asked us how we were doing. Family would ask me if I felt movement, which would cause me to panic all the time.

At a little over four months, when I started to feel movement, I had to hear the baby's heartbeat. At first, since it was still early in the pregnancy, the doctor couldn't get a heartbeat. He made us go to another room for a sonogram. He saw the heart pumping and said everything was fine.

We were always on edge.

We worried about Caitlyn the whole time. We went for numerous tests and every day hoped and prayed she would make it. Near the end we went every Monday and Friday to the doctors for Non-Stress tests and on Wednesday to the hospital for sonograms. A Biophysical Profile was taken every three weeks.

My children, now nearly nine and over six, were anxious, too, for their baby sister.

We wish we had had the same care with Sara as we had now with Caitlyn. If so, she would be here today.

The doctors wanted to do an amniocentesis at thirty six weeks and deliver Caitlyn a few days later so we wouldn't pass the mark of thirty seven and a half weeks when we lost Sara. However, the amniocentesis didn't go so well. The doctor had tapped blood and didn't know from where. We worried about what they hit. Also, since it was a 'bloody tap' they told me they shouldn't have used the specimen to check for lung maturity. Of course, when the tests came back the lungs were severely immature.

Two days and a lot of worry later, the doctor ended up delivering Caitlyn by C-section. It was a Friday evening and we went to the OB's office. My blood pressure had spiked. The doctor sent me to the hospital for observation. The doctor said I would be delivering this baby in about one hour. The anticipation was overwhelming. I cried as Caitlyn was being delivered. I wanted so much to see her alive. I wanted so much to hold her.

It was October 4, at seven P.M. Caitlyn was seven pounds, eleven ounces and healthy. Rich took pictures. Everyone in the room was so happy for us. We cried with joy and relief and grief for Sara.

A part of you feels so lucky and yet you feel sad. It was bittersweet.

Caitlyn still sleeps in my room every night right next to me or in my bed and she is twenty two months. I feared she would be a SIDS baby the first year. I always checked her breathing when she slept. A part of you always worries you will lose again.

Now we are pregnant with our fifth. I'm thirty three weeks pregnant and the sonograms have shown it's a boy. The kids are thrilled and already have a name picked out for him, Anthony. We are grateful and happy, but always wish we had our Sara, also. We feel as though she is watching over us and sent us Caitlyn and the new baby.

I really do feel so lucky to be a mom. Rich and I worry about this pregnancy also and have gone for many tests and already had one scary run to the hospital. I have about four and a half weeks to go and the closer I get, the more I cry for Sara. The more I think about her, the more I long for her.

I worry the same as I did with Caitlyn's pregnancy. If the baby is resting, I have to make him move or I panic. We can't wait for him to be here.

As with Caitlyn, I won't dare buy an outfit, bottle, or get the cradle ready. I will not accept any gifts prior to Anthony's delivery as I did the same for Caitlyn.

I hope our story provides support and encouragement to those who have been through this pain and sorrow. We've been very blessed to have other children and Sara will always be a very special part of our family. She will never be forgotten. We hope she knows how much we love her and how much we miss her every day of our lives.

We lost hope shortly after we lost Sara. I felt I would never conceive, that something was dreadfully wrong with me since my baby died inside of me and I couldn't save her. Patience, prayer and hope and family helped us along.

DONNA

Stephanie, Our Little Angel

One more day, one more time. One more sunset,
maybe I'd be satisfied.
But then again, I know what it would do.
Leave me wishing still, for one more day with you.
"One More Day" written by Steven Dale Jones and Bobby Tomberlin

Ray and I were married two years when we decided we were ready to start a family. We had a nice house on Long Island, and had well paying, stable jobs. I worked as a secretary in a church office and Ray was a power plant engineer. For the most part, Ray and I were very healthy and I did everything I was supposed to do: be off the pill for three months, take prenatal vitamins one month prior, cut out caffeine. I even had Ray wearing boxer shorts and taking a vitamin, too. We took one last couple trip for our second anniversary because we knew it would be a while before we would be able to do it again.

We started trying to get pregnant the month after our vacation and I was a fanatic about it. We tried every other day, and when the date I should've gotten my period came and it didn't begin, I didn't think too much of it. For three days I waited. I didn't want to believe I was pregnant, and on the first try, no less!

I kept telling myself I was just late. My best friend, who was pregnant with her second child, convinced me to buy a home pregnancy test. I bought a two-pack just in case the first one didn't work. The instructions said to use morning's first urine but I couldn't wait. I peed into a cup and inserted the tip of the tester in it and although the box tells you to wait one minute for an accurate result, the second line came up for positive before I could even pull up my pants!

I kept looking at the box to make sure two lines really meant, "You're pregnant." Ray was sitting on the couch when I came out of the bathroom and I told him the test was positive. He didn't believe me! He said I must have not done it right...but how can you mess up a pregnancy test? Good thing I bought a two-pack because I used it the next morning to satisfy my husband's disbelief.

He was very disappointed it happened on the first try; he thought we couldn't have more 'practice.' We saw my doctor that week and had a blood test to confirm. My due date was September 3, 2001. Labor Day, how ironic!

Since we found out our news a few days after Christmas, we kept it a secret from my family until we saw them the day before New Year's. I taped the pregnancy test inside of a box and gave it to my mother to open. I addressed it to Grandma and Grandpa, which didn't throw my mother off since we already had a dog and already called my parents by those names. When she opened it, she was speechless and looking at it because she couldn't figure out what it was at first and then she yelled, "You're pregnant!" It would be their first grandchild.

The nausea began in a couple of weeks and lasted all day. I tried all the things recommended: soda, crackers. Nothing worked. After a week of feeling like this, I'd had enough and got those wristbands for when you feel seasick or carsick and I don't know if it was mind over matter, but the nausea stopped within twenty minutes and I never took them off until my first trimester was over!

The second trimester was great. I wasn't tired anymore. I wanted to find out the sex of the baby so we could plan how the room would look and what kind of bedding we would register for. We didn't want neutral colors. Ray and I wanted it to be either blue or pink.

When it came time for our level II sonogram, the technician tried to see what it was, but the legs were crossed. I was so upset, but my doctor scheduled another sonogram because they weren't able to see all four chambers of the heart. At the next test, there was a good view of the heart and the lips and then we got a nice butt view with the legs apart and it showed signs of being a little girl.

We went right away to Toys R Us and Ray picked out a Baby Mickey doll for her and a toy steering wheel with sounds and lights. Ray likes racing cars, so this was right up his alley!

The next few days we went back and forth with our favorite names, and Ray's favorite was Stephanie. At first I wasn't too crazy about it, but the more I said it and referred to my belly as "Stephanie," the more I began to love it. Her middle name would be Eleanor for Ray's grandmother who had recently passed away.

During the third trimester I suffered from severe leg cramps at night. It was in the middle of summer and I was hot and miserable. I was getting big and Stephanie was pushing up into my chest. I found it hard to breathe and the humidity made it worse.

When I was seven months along, my family threw a baby shower. My sister-in-law took me out shopping and we were supposed to go to this restaurant for lunch. While I had a hunch this was the day, when I walked into the place and saw all those people who came to celebrate this baby and me, I was still surprised. We got everything we could possibly need and more.

My due date came and went with no sign of labor. A week later, my doctor sent me for a sonogram and they found my amniotic fluid was a little low. The doctor examined me and said I was three centimeters dilated. I should go to the hospital.

Immediately, the butterflies began in my stomach. We checked into the hospital in late afternoon, September 10th. In labor and delivery I was asked all those personal questions, and hooked up to an IV and given that fashionable hospital gown to wear. Around eight P.M. the doctor came in and gave the OK to start Pitocin. Even though I was dilated, I wasn't feeling any contractions. Within an hour, I was feeling them right on top of each other.

The anesthesiologist gave me the epidural. I only had to endure the very strong contractions for about a half hour before I got it, and that helped me to get some rest.

My husband, being on night shift for the last few weeks, was wide-awake and watching TV. Around three A.M., the doctor came in and asked me how I was feeling. I was having this strange pressure feeling. She checked me; I was nine and a half centimeters dilated and ready to push.

An infant bed was wheeled in. I started pushing at three fifteen A.M., and was still pushing at five thirty A.M. when the doctor came in and made the decision to do a C-section. I was exhausted, my epidural had worn off and I felt everything, from contractions to very bad back pain from pushing for so long. I was wheeled into the operating room, given more epidural medication, and prepped for surgery. When Ray came in all dressed in his scrubs, I began to get nervous about whether everything was all right.

The surgery went well and Stephanie Eleanor was born at six minutes past six A.M. on September 11, 2001.

I was in my room when the news about the World Trade Center was broadcast. The nurse brought Stephanie in, all clean and fed, at eleven A.M. She was just a little thing at six pounds, eight ounces. She had long, skinny legs, beautiful long eyelashes like me, and the most beautiful face. I couldn't believe I was a mom. I watched TV and thought about all those people who were lost. All those parents who lost a child and all those children who lost a parent. At a time when so many people lost loved ones, my family and I rejoiced at the birth of our little angel.

Two weeks after she was born, Stephanie began to give me problems feeding. She would arch her back and turn her head away from the bottle. She also didn't sleep for long periods of time. When she was awake, she spent much of the time being irritable. At her next check-up, her pediatrician, Dr. Z, told me she probably just had gas and not to worry. This behavior went on and on and I never called the pediatrician back because being a new mother, I didn't want them to think I was neurotic. At six weeks we saw Dr. W. who didn't like the way she looked. Stephanie seemed very pale to him and he also didn't like that she hadn't gained weight, as she should have. She was finally sleeping better, and never woke at night for a bottle. Dr. W. referred us to a geneticist who didn't see anything wrong and referred us to a gastroenterologist who prescribed Zantac.

I had to wake her at night to try to feed her. When we saw the gastroenterologist Stephanie's feedings hadn't improved. She was hospitalized to put a feeding tube in her nose to begin continuous pump feedings at night. She was three months old.

When Stephanie was released from the hospital just before Christmas Eve, her nursery became a hospital room with a feeding pump, which I learned to operate, feeding bags and vials for medicine. She was put on a special formula that cannot be bought in any store and is very expensive. I also had to add a calorie booster to her formula.

I still had to try oral feedings and whatever she didn't finish had to be put into a vial and put through the tube in her nose. Since Stephanie was so behind in her skills, Early Intervention Services was called in and she began to receive physical therapy, feeding and speech therapy.

A nutritionist came twice a month, as did a nurse to weigh her. Three months passed and when her oral feedings still hadn't improved, she had an upper GI series which revealed an enlarged heart.

I followed-up with a cardiologist. On the day of the appointment, Ray had to work, so my mother came with us.

After the test at the cardiologist, my mother left, and the doctor came in. I was alone with Stephanie when he told me something was very wrong with her heart and to go straight to the hospital, for immediate admittance to Pediatric ICU for full work-up.

I was in shock because I remember asking him, "You want me to go *right now!?*" I was thinking, *I'll go home, pack a bag, come later with Ray*, but NO, he wanted me to go immediately. I called Ray at work and he left to meet us at the hospital.

When Stephanie and I got to the ICU, they put her in a hospital gown and hooked her up to all types of machines. The nurses asked me a lot of questions about her history. I remember feeling like I was having an out of body experience. I could hear myself answering, but I felt like I was floating above my head and watching myself responding. I found out later this behavior is very normal in this situation.

After a full work-up and ten days in the hospital, Stephanie was sent home and had to be on three heart medications. In just a couple of months of being a new mother, I became a nurse and had to learn really fast how to measure medications accurately so as to not overdose her.

I would remove the tube in her nose every two weeks and insert a new one in the other nostril. My friends and family didn't know how I could do it, but I told them, "What choice do I have?" She had to get nourishment. I couldn't be scared or grossed out by it. Stephanie depended on me to keep her from getting sicker.

Stephanie's life became a constant barrage of doctor's appointments and medications, and my life, as I had known it, became non-existent. Nothing in my life mattered anymore than finding out what was making my daughter so sick.

When her heart was stable enough, Stephanie went into the hospital for a third time to put a gastric tube directly into her stomach so she didn't have to have the awful one in her nose anymore.

We consulted a cardiologist at a hospital in Manhattan for a second opinion. She agreed with the initial diagnosis and referred us to their genetics department. I was very hesitant to see another geneticist, who, I felt, would again tell me they couldn't see anything wrong. But the cardiologist strongly urged me to call, so this got me thinking, *Maybe she knows something I don't*, so I decided to take Stephanie to their geneticist.

This geneticist took one look at her and based on her facial features, knew right away she had some sort of storage disorder. A full body x-ray confirmed what she had suspected. After more urine and blood tests, Ray and I were told our daughter had a terminal, genetic, metabolic disorder called Mucolipidosis Type II (aka I-cell disease).

Ray and I are carriers of this disease and unknowingly passed it on to her. *How could we do this to our child*? I thought. Although we had no way of knowing we were carriers until a child was affected, I never felt so guilty in my entire life! Stephanie was ten months old and we were told this disorder would continue to wreak havoc on her body.

She would cease to grow at two years and her problems with feedings would most likely continue. She would never walk, potty train or go to school. She would just get sicker over time until her death by the age of ten, although most children don't live beyond five or six years old. Death is usually from pneumonia or heart complications.

We were devastated.

Although we were told there was no permanent treatment or cure for this disease, a week after she was diagnosed, the geneticist called to say she had done some research and found a hospital in Minnesota who had been successful in treating children with this disease with a bone marrow transplant. It wasn't a cure, it would only, at best, slow the progression of the disease.

She spoke to the bone marrow transplant team at their hospital in Manhattan and the Director agreed to meet with us to discuss this procedure. Although this hospital hadn't treated Stephanie's specific disease, they had treated children with a similar storage disorder with a bone marrow transplant and were successful. We knew if we didn't try this transplant, Stephanie would just get sicker and suffer terribly until she died.

Ray was one hundred percent for it from the get-go, without even meeting the doctor, but I had a lot of questions and concerns. My major concern was I didn't want my daughter to be their guinea pig.

At our meeting, the procedure and all the risks involved were explained. Considering Stephanie's age, the doctor felt it was safer to do a cord blood transplant since an infant's blood would be more suitable and we had a better chance of finding a match.

We were to let the doctor know the following week what we wanted to do. It was a lot to comprehend and Ray and I didn't agree on a decision. He didn't want to think about the risk of death, he just wanted to try anything to make her better and if she died, then maybe it was for the best.

And I, well, while my brain understood this was my only way to give my daughter a chance at a better quality of life; my heart told me not to do it because I feared the worst. She could die during the transplant.

The disease had affected Stephanie's heart. Even though we got the OK from both cardiologists that her heart could withstand the toxic chemotherapy drugs given to her, I wasn't one hundred percent convinced this was the right thing to do. But we had no other options, and if we *didn't* do it, a part of me didn't want to spend the rest of my life wondering if it would've worked for her. So after much deliberation, I hesitantly agreed to go ahead with the transplant.

While this grim news and plans for a long hospitalization hovered over our heads, we went ahead with our plans for a big party for Stephanie's first birthday. All her family and friends came out to celebrate her life and she got lots of presents and well wishes. In another month, she would be going into the hospital for the biggest fight of her life!

Stephanie was thirteen months old when she went into the hospital for the fourth and, unbeknownst to all of us, her final time. She had to have surgery to insert a port into her chest so all the medications would be given through there instead of her being pricked all the time. She got through the insertion procedure well and began chemotherapy the next day. She was doing very well with the chemotherapy, always had a smile throughout the entire process.

On October 21, the fourth day of chemotherapy, Stephanie awoke very distressed after a drug infusion. I sat her up and tried to soothe her as she screamed and jerked her body in such obvious pain. I called for a nurse who came in and sent for the on-call doctor.

As Stephanie sat there crying, she reached out her hand and reached for my shoulder and as I looked into her eyes, I swear she was trying to say,

Mommy, help me, I'm scared. After the nurse left and I laid her down in the bed, she jerked her body and screamed again. When I looked down at her stomach, her shirt had blood on it and when I pulled up her shirt, blood was seeping out from around the g-tube in her stomach. I panicked and ran out of the room screaming, "Help me!" The nurses came running.

In a matter of minutes Stephanie began to have trouble breathing and went into cardiac arrest. I found myself alone as I watched my daughter slip away right in front of my eyes, a sight I will never forget.

I heard the words "Child in cardiac arrest." Doctors from ICU came running into the room and started working on her, trying to bring her back.

The nurse took me to a lounge to wait. The doctor finally came in and I remember thinking he's going to tell me she'll be transferred to ICU for closer monitoring. Instead he told me they did everything they could, but she didn't make it.

I buried my head in the nurse's arm, sobbing. My worst fear had come true. She was dead.

She would never receive the perfectly matched cord blood and she would never have the chance to see if the transplant would have worked. Right then, all my plans and dreams for her and for us were gone forever.

One of the social workers called Ray at home, but got the answering machine and left a message asking him to call the hospital. He was home sleeping and heard the machine click off, so when he heard the message he called right back. I got on the phone with him and his first words were, "Is she dead?" and I said, "Yes," but he already knew she was gone. As he cried, I couldn't believe how calm I was. I told him to call my parents and come to the hospital together. I didn't want him driving alone.

The trip to the hospital was about an hour and a half. My husband told me later the drive felt like "forever."

A staff member took me back to the room. Stephanie was lying in bed, her eyes closed, looking so peaceful. I just remember making sure she was covered with her blanket because she was so cold already. The nurses cut a little hair from her head and made a clay mold of her foot and they put together a memory box for me to take home.

Ray and my parents showed up and we stayed with Stephanie, each taking turns holding her. I held her and sang her favorite song, *The Itsy Bitsy Spider.*

The doctor finally came after midnight to pronounce her so the death certificate says her day of death is October 22, when in reality she died at eleven fifty P.M. on October 21. I feel like I mourn her death for two days instead of one.

It was three A.M. when I felt I had to let her go so they could get her ready for us to bury her. We all gave our last kisses goodbye and we left. I took home the blanket they had wrapped her in and I held it the whole ride home. I walked into the hospital holding my child and left early another morning without her in my arms.

I felt I was no longer a mother and we were no longer a family.

I was overwhelmed with grief and guilt.

I blamed myself for her death because I should've listened to my heart and not gone through with the transplant. I felt I should've been smart enough to know her heart was just too weak and couldn't withstand the treatment. Ray tried to make me feel better by reminding me if we didn't do this transplant she would just get sicker and it wouldn't be fair to her, but I just couldn't see it his way.

I was selfish and felt I would take care of her as I'd been doing all along. While I know it would have been very hard to see her that way, I felt we could have had more time to take her places, like Disney World and we could have had plenty of time to say goodbye. I was more heartbroken over the loss of her in my life than to think about what her life would've been like had we not done the transplant.

I felt I'd failed Stephanie and my family, especially my father, who took Stephanie's death the hardest. I was angry with myself and angry with my husband and my family for convincing me to do the transplant.

The day we buried our daughter was the hardest thing I've ever had to endure in my life. When I left the cemetery, I broke down crying, "I don't want to leave my baby here!"

The whole restaurant event after the funeral was a blur. I just wanted to go home and go to bed and never come out. Stephanie was the love of my life. She had a lot of special needs I took care of, and not doing them anymore left me helpless, depressed and alone.

Ray and I had to get away, so we went to Pennsylvania, back to the place we went for our last trip before we decided to get pregnant. I made a promise to myself that I wouldn't let her death keep me from continuing with my life and getting out of bed in the morning.

The week after we came back I returned to my part-time job. It was hard because Stephanie came with me every day but everyone at work was very supportive, as they had been the whole time she was sick, when I was out so often to be with her in the hospital or leave early for doctor appointments.

Lots of people just didn't know what to say to me and told me so. Part of me didn't want them to say anything because I didn't want to start crying in front of them.

While work kept my mind occupied for the morning, I spent many afternoons shopping because I couldn't bear to be home alone. The house was too quiet!

Sleeping was torture; every time I closed my eyes I relived the night she died. I just couldn't get those moments out of my head. I spent many nights holding her blanket so I could smell her and feel like she was still here.

I read every book on loss of a child I could get my hands on. It felt so good to know the way I felt was perfectly normal and it wouldn't last forever. I also looked into support groups and was disappointed we would have to wait three months after her death to go to one. I couldn't understand *why*? I needed help now, not later! When the wait was up, I found a support group through a hospital in our area that met once a week for six weeks.

Ray didn't feel the need to go because, from the moment she died, he was at peace with it and felt she was in a better place, free from the pain of her disease. He only went for me, for which I was thankful.

Our first meeting was held four and a half months after Stephanie died. We met a lot of other people going through the same anger, grief and loneliness. For the first time in months, I felt like I wasn't alone! While it was very painful to tell the story of how she died all over again, it felt good to let it out.

We all cried and yelled and got a lot of our frustrations and feelings out. After it ended, Ray and I went to a monthly drop-in group called The Guardian Angel Perinatal Support Group (GAPS, part of the National SHARE program), led by Martha, a bereaved mom herself and an LPN with training in perinatal bereavement. It really does help to have other people around you who know exactly what you are going through and how you feel because no one, not family and not friends, could possibly know.

I began to see a therapist who helped me to let go of some of the guilt, but some days it still sneaks up on me. For right now, I'm still trying to adjust to our new lives, a life forever changed since the loss of Stephanie. Vacations aren't the same, holidays aren't the same...I'M NOT THE SAME! I used to be afraid of dying and now I'm not, because I know she will be waiting for me with her big beautiful smile. Here on earth, I know she is around my family and me always.

To keep her memory alive, I have a special place in the house where I have pictures of her and angel figurines. The most memorable thing I did was take all the video footage of her short life and professionally preserve it for my family with pictures of Stephanie in the beginning and a music montage at the end recapping the entire video. It came out wonderfully and I watch it often.

Emily, Our Second Chance

The grand essentials of happiness are: something to do,
something to love, and something to hope for.
Allan K. Chalmers

The day after we buried Stephanie, Ray said to me if I wanted to try again tomorrow, he would say yes. I was shocked, considering he was the one who wanted to wait two years for the first child. To hear him say yes really made me see how much Stephanie meant to him and how much he missed her, too.

I knew I didn't want to wait a year to get pregnant, like all the books I read said I should. A year felt like an eternity and my biological clock was ticking. Stephanie was laid out on my thirtieth birthday, and while people laughed at me when I told them this, her death made me feel old.

Thanksgiving and Christmas were coming up and I felt we should wait until after the holidays to try again since it would be our first holidays without Stephanie. They proved to be a tough test of my emotions, but we got through them and I was proud of that littlest accomplishment. We remembered Stephanie on those days with the entire family going to the cemetery and releasing balloons. We each wrote a special message on the balloons and let them go and watched them disappear into the clouds as if Stephanie had plucked them right out of the sky. We continue to do this every holiday and for her birthday.

Even though I was excited about the thought of holding another child in my arms, it wouldn't be an easy road since the disorder Stephanie had was genetic and there was a one in four chance of it happening again in future pregnancies.

While I tried to see the brighter side of it . . . the seventy-five percent chance of it *not* happening, I couldn't think about that because we already had one child who *didn't* fall into that seventy-five percent range, so if it happened once, it could happen again.

I would have to undergo prenatal testing during the pregnancy to see if this baby had the disorder. We had already decided if the child did have the disorder, we would terminate the pregnancy because we couldn't bear the thought of burying another child, nor could we put a child through the suffering and pain this disorder can cause, knowing in the end, our child would die.

This was another reason why I didn't want to wait forever to try again because if we had to terminate, I knew we would have to wait a few months after to try again.

We tried in January 2003, and again got pregnant on the first try. I bought a home pregnancy test and did it while Ray was at work. It was the week before Valentine's Day and I bought my husband an early card and taped the positive pregnancy test inside of it. He saw it and got this big smile on his face. While I was happy about being a mother again, I was terrified at the thought, *would this child be one I would be able to keep*? I tried to be positive, but it was hard.

So many things ran through my head and made this pregnancy mentally stressful. I felt if this child wasn't a girl, I didn't know if I would love it the way I loved Stephanie. Sometimes, I thought even if I had a little girl, I wouldn't want to bond with her because I would miss Stephanie too much. I felt I failed Stephanie and was a horrible mother, so how could I be a mother to another child? Because I couldn't feed Stephanie like a normal baby, I questioned my ability to care for another child, and a healthy one. I didn't think I would know what to do.

I also felt people would think I was forgetting about Stephanie if I got pregnant too soon after her death. We decided to only tell my parents until after all the tests were done. They were very happy for us. When my father hugged me and said, "Thank you," I knew we made the right decision to get pregnant now.

In my first trimester, I felt great physically. I had some nausea in the beginning, but nothing like I did with Stephanie. Mentally though, this pregnancy took its toll. I dreaded every doctor's appointment wondering if they would find something wrong.

I left Martha's support group because hearing all the women's stories of miscarriages and stillborns so late in their pregnancies made me even more scared. Part of me felt God didn't want me to be a mother and even though this baby was healthy, he would make it so I couldn't have her, either.

I began to read again and looked for books on subsequent pregnancies after the loss of child. I was so afraid I wasn't going to bond or love this baby the way I loved Stephanie. I didn't think a healthy baby would need me the way Stephanie did. The books helped me to see all these feelings were perfectly normal. I just couldn't bring myself to be excited about being pregnant as I was the first time.

When I went for my second month checkup, I began to make plans for the prenatal test, CVS, to be done. We decided to do it because it could be done between ten and twelve weeks instead of waiting for an amniocentesis, which is done later. Ray and I went to the same hospital where Stephanie died and the same genetics department where we were told Stephanie's diagnosis. That was hard, but I tried not to think about it.

It would be over a week before we would knew the results. On the tenth day, the doctor called and said this baby tested negative for the disorder. We were so relieved. Chromosome tests were also normal and we found out it was a girl.

After the good news, I felt I could be excited about being pregnant. We felt we could tell everyone we were going to have another baby and everyone was happy for us.

Ever since I was pregnant the first time I loved the name Emily, so since Ray had chosen Stephanie's name, I felt it only fair I choose this baby's name. Our new daughter's name would be Emily Rose.

We decided to keep the nursery the same. One of the hardest things I had to do was get Stephanie's baby clothes out of storage. I wondered if I would cry each time I dressed Emily in the morning, seeing her wearing her sister's clothes. Those boxes stayed in the nursery for weeks before I could bring myself to go through them.

One dress I insisted Emily not wear was Stephanie's first birthday outfit. It would go into a shadow-box with some of her other special things. I couldn't bring myself to take down Stephanie's name plaque off the nursery wall or other knickknacks with her name, never to be looked at again. To this day, she has her own little shelf with special things and her picture. I felt it was and always would be her room because she never was old enough to move out of it. I felt she would be my baby forever!

My second and third trimesters didn't go well. I suffered from pelvic pressure so severe I could barely walk. And the bigger I got, the worse the pain became. Blood tests showed I was anemic.

When I was thirty six weeks along, I began cramping much like when I was pregnant with Stephanie. This was on September 10th, the day before Stephanie was born. I was so afraid I was having labor pains and this baby would be born on her birthday and I wanted that day to be only hers. I went to the doctor and he put me on partial bed rest for the last month. The cramping was due to dehydration, so I had to drink a lot of fluids. This seemed to be a problem for me when I was pregnant...keeping hydrated!

We decided to do a repeat C-section. We planned it for October 10th. A week before, the doctor moved it to October 8th, which was fine with me because I just wanted Emily to be here. It had been a long nine months. This would be extra special since it was also my grandmother's birthday.

We were at the hospital at six A.M. I got into my hospital gown and my IV was inserted and we waited and watched the sun come up. At eight A.M., I walked down the hall to the surgery room. Ray came in wearing his scrubs and I began to cry when I saw him because then I knew this was it, there was no turning back now. The surgery went well and Emily was born at eight sixteen A.M. with all ten fingers and toes. The moment was so bittersweet.

I cried when I saw her beautiful face. The nurse knew of my loss, and when she saw Emily she pointed out her top lip, which was heart-shaped. The nurse said it meant Stephanie had kissed her on the way out. It was love at first sight, and I bonded with Emily right away. Feeding her with a bottle was a delight; I didn't want anyone else to do it. The second night we were in the hospital, I even had the nurse bring her to me for the middle of the night feeding so I could experience what it was like, since I didn't have that with Stephanie. I never thought I would be so excited about having to get up in the middle of the night for a feeding!

The first few months were very hard emotionally and physically trying to adjust to feedings, sleepless nights and having an infant in the house again. But Emily was a wonderful distraction because I didn't dwell on Stephanie's death as much.

I loved holding her and when she fell asleep in my arms, I didn't want to put her down.

Still, I questioned my ability to be a mother every single day. I cried a lot and called my best friend for advice all the time. I wasn't a neurotic, first-time mother with Stephanie, but this time I felt like I was. I called the pediatrician all the time when Emily was an infant. Even though Emily was thriving I dreaded the pediatrician visits, hoping she had gained weight.

I felt like I needed to make up for lost time and I try to do all the things with Emily I couldn't do with Stephanie. I got Emily's ears pierced. I enrolled her in swimming lessons for the two of us, which was very special bonding time. We also joined a Mommy'n'Me class, which she loves and I love doing with her. As a family, we've taken her to the aquarium and the zoo and we plan to take her to Disney World next year for Christmas since as Ray says, "Stephanie was never able to go." I know he is also trying to give Emily everything he would've given to Stephanie had he been given the chance.

Because Stephanie wasn't very mobile and was very content in her jumper or her booster seat, Emily has presented a challenge for me. When she was nine months old, she began to crawl and everywhere I went she followed. Privacy became a thing of the past and so did my sanity. She began to pull herself up on everything and because she wasn't quite steady yet, she sustained quite a few bumps and bruises. I think it hurt me more than her to see her fall.

I love holding and rocking her to sleep at night. When Emily falls sound asleep in my arms, I find myself reminiscing about holding Stephanie the night she passed away, so still, and it brings tears to my eyes.

Emily loves to hear herself talk and she makes my husband and me laugh all the time with her antics. But the very best is when Emily says "Mama," which I never got to hear Stephanie say.

I still question how much formula/milk to give her and how often. This is my biggest fear. I'm a fanatic about her finishing her bottles. I don't care as much if she doesn't finish her food, as long as she finishes her bottle, since Stephanie's nutritionist told me the formula was more important than food for weight gain and nutrition. Everyone told me feedings would be easier with a healthy child, but I found it to be more stressful than it was with Stephanie.

I'm trying to tell myself Emily knows when she is hungry or full and if I get agitated during feedings, she will sense it and it won't be good for her. Emily is almost a year old now, healthy, as far I know, and walking everywhere.

Thanks to medication, my nerves have finally started to calm down. This has helped me to realize, if she doesn't finish her bottle, I don't freak out. I just want to cherish every second with Emily since I know how fast it can all be taken away.

Over the last few months she has begun to remind me so much of Stephanie. When she smiles, she looks so much like her. She has her blue eyes, the same smile and happy personality as Stephanie did. I have a picture frame in the house with pictures of Emily and Stephanie in it and sometimes when I walk by and look at it, I have to look twice because I wonder which one it's a picture of. I cannot count how many times I've been told how beautiful Emily is. It makes me so happy and proud that I helped bring another child into this world; Emily makes me and other people have a smile on our faces.

Emily comes with us to the cemetery to visit Stephanie and we say her name to her all the time and show her pictures. A part of me feels like Emily already knows her because when she was an infant, I showed her a picture of Stephanie and she didn't take her eyes off of it. I got goose bumps.

I truly believe Stephanie is Emily's guardian angel and is watching over her. I know she is looking down on us and she is looking out for Emily. I love telling Emily she has a big sister and I can't wait until she is old enough to know all about her.

My focus right now is on being Emily's mommy and giving to her everything we couldn't give Stephanie. I know Stephanie is making my grandparents very happy in heaven as she had made us here on earth. Emily has filled a void in the family's heart. They all adore her and we have all begun to slowly heal from the loss of Stephanie.

We would love to have one more child, and look forward to trying again in the next year or so. But for now, I'm enjoying having my little girl back in my arms again and my second chance at being a mother and a family.

PEACEFUL TRANSITIONS

What the caterpillar calls the end of the world, the Master calls a butterfly.
Illusions Richard Bach

When Amy approached me to write the summation to her book, I was honored. As a practicing Social Worker, I have worked with many families over the past fourteen years who have experienced the loss of a baby. Seven years ago, a young mother expecting twins had the misfortune of losing one of her babies. She was devastated and even more so when she discovered there were no formal support groups at the hospital for her to process her grief. She set up a fund in honor of her son, Tyler Ford Bialek. The fund was used to establish support groups for perinatal loss. My colleagues and I developed the Perinatal Bereavement Program for Winthrop University Hospital, in Mineola, NY. This program has been a lifeline for many couples struggling with the pain of loss. The program ultimately expanded to include groups for those who interrupted a much-wanted pregnancy due to anomalies. The last group to form was the SPALS group, (subsequent pregnancy after a loss). There have been many new friendships formed and a community of families dedicated to preserving the memory of their babies as well as offering support to one another.

The loss of a baby is probably the single most devastating event a couple/family can experience. No one is ever prepared to lose their baby and no one is prepared to deal with all the emotions that come with loss. The prenatal books prepare you for life, but they don't focus on loss and if they do, it's usually a tiny section at the back of the book.

If you're pregnant for the first time it's utter bliss, there's a euphoria that comes over you as if you have achieved the unachievable, you are special because you are carrying precious cargo. It's a new life and you're responsible for bringing it into the world. This new little baby will have his or her own distinct personality. The baby's future will already be mentally mapped out. There will be the first of everything. The first smile, the first tooth, the first steps, the play dates, the first day of school, birthday parties and the list goes on and on. But once you experience the loss of your pregnancy, everything changes.

The world as you knew it no longer exits and nothing seems to make any sense. Family and friends don't know what to say to you. Some say nothing and pretend nothing happened and some feel compelled to "fix you" by saying something profound or trying to distract you from your pain. Unless they've been there, no words or actions can heal the pain a couple feels.

From the moments in labor and delivery when the ultimate cruelty is realized, the birth is a silent one. This was not in the plan and as days and weeks pass, the grief process is relentless. It's one wave after another of crashing emotions pounding on a weakened spirit. The cruelty of not having your baby does not stop there but is the constant reminder of who is missing in your family. Instead of going through all the firsts with a living baby you are now going through all the firsts of losing one. You have now entered the group that no one wants to belong to.

It has been my experience that when a couple experiences a loss of a baby the journey of grief can be a difficult one. Since men and women grieve very differently it's so important to keep the lines of communication open. This is not the time for one partner to protect the other, however, it's a time for each of them to sit in the midst of their pain and reach out to one another. Sitting with your pain allows you to move to another phase of grief. Those who are clever and nicely package their pain away...well, at some point down the road the package starts to unwrap, and when that happens it's much more difficult to control the emotions or reactions to them. Allow yourself the feeling and see where the journey takes you. If you stop the feelings, you also stop the journey.

Following couples from the loss of their baby to the subsequent pregnancy is quite challenging. Anxiety and fear become your companions in the subsequent pregnancy. What can go wrong will go wrong, or so you are convinced. Bonding with the new pregnancy and baby growing within becomes more difficult. Your fear holds you back; you already know bad things do happen because they've happened to you. You're not so bold in announcing you're pregnant again and at times you may wish you could be invisible. The SPALS group has been one of the most beneficial groups formed. This group focuses on the issues grieving parents face when they become pregnant again. The primary thing is they are not alone with their fears and anxieties.

One of my most precious memories is with a couple who joined our first SPALS group. The first group consisted of two couples who experienced the loss of their first baby. Both were to deliver daughters and both girls were born still at term. Though the two couples were not in the same grief group, they met each other at a Reunion Group. When they both became pregnant with the subsequent pregnancy the anxiety they felt was overwhelming. The SPALS group met twice a month, the first and third Wednesdays. The two couples would meet diligently, not allowing anything to get in the way. The group became their lifeline to remaining sane. In the months that followed, the couples focused on all the testing they were undergoing and the daily anxiety attacks they were experiencing. The looks, from family and friends speculating whether there was a new pregnancy, but would not dare to ask, added undue stress. They also focused on how the new pregnancy did not make the grief process go away, and yet expressed fear about forgetting the memory of their first baby when the new baby arrived. At twenty weeks both couples wanted to know the sex of their baby. The thought of waiting for a surprise was out of the question.

The feeling of being out of control was not one they wanted to visit again. Though the reality is, no matter how much control you think you have, you quickly find out how much control you really don't have. Both couples were expecting baby boys. The wounds of grief opened again at this time. On some level, though they knew this was a "new" pregnancy and a "new" baby the harsh reality that they weren't getting the baby they lost was becoming clear. As the pregnancies continued so did the anxiety.

One of the couples was delivering at my hospital. They asked if I would be present at the birth of their son. I must admit, it was the most wonderful gift anyone has ever given me. As a Social Worker, no one ever calls you when things are going well. The birth of Joseph would be one of the single most precious experiences of my life.

I'll never forget getting the phone call that it was time to go. Sitting with Rosemarie and Don for hours in labor and delivery, I got to know them on a different level. I wasn't just the therapist or the facilitator at that moment, I was a friend. I was invited into a very private and personal moment that would define the rest of their lives. As Rosemarie's labor intensified, I realized how important it was to have the volume of the fetal monitor turned on. The sound of the baby's heartbeat was a new sound and the only sound that communicated the baby was alive. There was constant reassurance that things were OK and even occasional comedy to lighten things up. On the nightstand there was a small framed picture of their first baby, Olivia. They made sure that no one would forget that Joseph had an older sister. It was finally time and on July 29, 2003 at two twenty two A.M., Joseph was born! He entered the world crying and kicking! It was such an emotional experience and one I will cherish always. Since Joseph's birth I have had the joy of witnessing the births of several other babies all of which were the result of a subsequent pregnancy after a loss. Joseph, George and Amanda will always hold a special place in my heart.

All the feelings you are feeling are normal and validated by the stories you have just read. Remember, the journey is a long one and though it may pause at times, it's really one that's ongoing. No matter how many subsequent pregnancies you go on to have, the memory of the baby that was wanted, wished for and lost, will always be present, and that's OK. The goal is to find a new "normal."

Memorializing your baby is a significant way of preserving the memory of your baby. Many of the families I have worked with have been very creative in how they honored their babies. Some families planted a garden or tree in their backyard. Others made financial donations to a perinatal bereavement fund. Some became advocates in the area of perinatal loss while others released balloons or tossed a message in a bottle in the ocean, and every one of the chapters in this book is in memory of a precious baby. The ways of memorializing are endless. You need to find something that feels right for you.

I wish you peace on your journey.
Anna Orologio, LMSW

EPILOGUE

Where there is great love there are always miracles.
Death Comes for the Archbishop, Willa Cather

The authors have gone through some very personal challenges. What kept us going isn't any secret recipe I can share. For some of us, it was perseverance, for others, prayer. All of us found out how to mourn in the midst of the chaos of our lives. We learned who our supporters were, and who they were not. We argued with spouses, and learned how to forgive ourselves. Luckily, all of our marriages survived. Our inner strength and faith was tested.

In coping through our subsequent pregnancies, some of us had baby showers and attended birthing classes again. For others, the pain and fear prohibited such activities. Some included their losses on their birth announcements as a way of honoring our lost children.

Three of us went on to have additional pregnancies, our SSPALS – subsequent SPALS. Two of us are currently pregnant again. We've enjoyed the milestones our children have brought to us, and continue to memorialize our losses in many ways.

Public speaking has been helpful for many. We've shared our experiences at "reunion groups," both pregnancy loss groups and pregnancy after loss groups. I've spoken at loss groups since my daughter was two months old—nineteen months after I lost Solomon. And now when I attend, there are group graduates there whom I've spoken to, shared with and cried with. To me that is a wonderful gift, seeing I made a difference in helping some others on their journeys, and that they, too, are making a difference.

The advent of the Internet has been a wonderful tool for many of us. We posted on support groups, created memorial websites and lit virtual candles to honor our children.

Memorial conferences have occurred, with speakers who are experts in the field of pregnancy and loss as well as parents, experts of their own experiences. Some of us have been behind the scenes as planners.

A memorial quilt was assembled. Parents were asked to contribute fabric squares memorializing their losses. The squares were assembled into a quilt that is now part of Winthrop University Hospital. Photos, notes, decorations, all have become part of the quilt.

As time passes, we find ourselves more and more engaged in moving forward and on with our lives. Some of our connections to each other remain and we are there to share all the ups and downs of parenthood. Spouses, children, family, jobs—there are a myriad of things to be attended to. And on our anniversaries, we remember with sadness, what could have been.

RESOURCES

This resource list is just a sampling of what is available. Please speak with your doctor or other medical professional for further suggestions.

Books

A Silent Love: Personal Stories of Coming to Terms with Miscarriage, Adrienne Ryan. Marlowe and Company, 2001.

A Silent Sorrow: Pregnancy Loss; Guidance and Support for You and Your Family, Ingrid Kohn, Perry-Lynn Moffitt, Isabelle A. Wilkins. Routledge; 2nd edition, 2000.

A Woman Doctor's Guide to Miscarriage: Essential Facts and Up-To-The Minute Information on Coping With Pregnancy Loss and Trying Again, Lynn Friedman, Irene Daria, Laurie Abkemeier (Editor), Arene Daria. Hyperion, 1996.

An Empty Cradle, a Full Heart: Reflections for Mothers and Fathers After Miscarriage, Stillbirth, or Infant Death, Christine O'Keeffe Lafser, Phyllis Tickle. Loyola Press, 1998.

Another Baby? Maybe . . ., Sherokee Ilse and Maribeth Wilder Doerr. Wintergreen Press, Maple Plain MN. Available from A Place to Remember, (800) 631-0973. 1996.

Coming to Term: A Father's Story of Birth, Loss, and Survival, William H. Woodwell, Jr. University Press of Mississippi, 2001.

Days in Waiting: A Guide to Surviving Pregnancy Bedrest, Mary Ann McCann. Deruyter-Nelson Publications, 1999.

Empty Arms: Coping After Miscarriage, Stillbirth and Infant Death. Sherokee Ilse (Editor). Wintergreen Press, Maple Plain MN. Available from A Place to Remember, (800) 631-0973. 1982/2002.

Empty Cradle, Broken Heart: Surviving the Death of Your Baby, Deborah L. Davis, PhD. Fulcrum Publishing; Revised edition, 1996.

Help, Comfort and Hope After Losing Your Baby in Pregnancy or the First Year, Hannah Lothrop. Perseus Publishing, 1997/2004.

Life Touches Life: A Mother's Story of Stillbirth and Healing, Lorraine Ash. New Sage Press, 2004.

Miscarriage: A Man's Book, Rick Wheat. The Centering Corporation, 1995.

Miscarriage: Women Sharing from the Heart, Marie Allen, Ph.D. & Shelly Marks, MS. John Wiley & Sons, 1993.

Mommy, Please Don't Cry: There Are No Tears in Heaven, Linda DeYmaz. Multnomah Gifts, 2003.

Our Stories of Miscarriage: Healing With Words, Rachel Faldet and Karen Fitton. Fairview Press, 1997.

Parenthood Lost: Healing the Pain after Miscarriage, Stillbirth, and Infant Death, Michael Berman, MD. Greenwood Press, 2000.

Pregnancy After Loss: A Guide to Pregnancy After a Miscarriage, Stillbirth or Infant Death, Carol Cirulli Lanham. Berkeley Publishing Group, 1999.

Still to be Born: A Guide for Bereaved Parents Who are Making Decisions About Their Future, Pat Schwiebert, RN and Paul Kirk, MD. Perinatal Loss, Portland, OR. Available from A Place to Remember, 1885 University Avenue, Saint Paul, MN 55104, (800) 631-0973. 1989.

Taking Charge of Your Fertility by Toni Weschler. HarperCollins, Revised 2001.

The Shadow of an Angel - Diary of a Subsequent Pregnancy Following a Neonatal Loss, Marion Cohen. Liberal Press, PO Box 160361, Los Colinas, TX 75016, 1986.

Trying Again: A Guide to Pregnancy After Miscarriage, Stillbirth, and Infant Loss, Ann Douglas, John R. Sussman, M.D. Taylor Publications, 2000.

Unspeakable Losses: Healing from Miscarriage, Abortion and Other Pregnancy Loss, by Kim Kluger-Bell. HarperCollins, 2000.

When Hello Means Goodbye: A Guide for Parents Whose Child Dies Before Birth, at Birth, or Shortly After Birth, Pat Schwiebert, RN and Paul Kirk, MD. Perinatal Loss, 1998.

Organizations and Websites
(advocacy, memorial items, resources, support)

❖ www.AMENDInc.com
AMEND, Inc. is a lay group of volunteers which offers a listening ear, a strong shoulder, and a compassionate heart to aid mothers and fathers as they experience normal grief following a neonatal death or miscarriage. The volunteer counselors, who have all experienced similar deaths, are available to listen, to understand, and to give moral support to grieving parents.

AMEND
P.O. Box 20260
Wichita, Kansas 67208-1260
Phone 316-268-8441
Email: info@amendinc.com

❖ www.APlaceToRemember.com
A Place To Remember is committed to publishing and providing uplifting support materials and resources for those who have been touched by a crisis in pregnancy or the death of a baby.

A Place To Remember
1885 University Avenue, Suite 110
St. Paul MN 55104
Phone: 800-631-0973 Fax 651-645-4780

❖ www.BereavedParentsUSA.org
Bereaved Parents of the USA (BP/USA) is a national non-profit self-help group that offers support, understanding, compassion and hope to bereaved parents, grandparents and siblings struggling to rebuild their lives after the death of their children, grandchildren or siblings.

Bereaved Parents USA
P.O. Box 95
Park Forest, Illinois 60466
Phone: 708-748-7866

❖ www.BereavementServices.org
Bereavement Services is the leading national and international provider of bereavement training and support services for professionals who care for bereaved families.

Bereavement Services
Gundersen Lutheran Medical Foundation
1900 South Avenue
La Crosse, WI 54601
Phone: 608-775-4747 or 800-362-9567 ext. 54747   Fax 608-775-5137
Email: info@bereavementservices.org

❖ www.CenteringCorp.com
The Centering Corporation is a non-profit organization dedicated to providing education and resources for the bereaved.

The Centering Corporation
1531 N. Saddle Creek Rd

Omaha, NE 68104-5064

Phone: 402-553-1200

E-mail: J1200@aol.com

❖ www.Climb-Support.org

CLIMB (Center for Loss in Multiple Birth) serves families and others throughout the United States, Canada and beyond. They provide parent-to-parent support for all who have experienced the death of one or more twins or higher multiple birth children at any time from conception through birth, infancy and early childhood.

Center for Loss in Multiple Birth (CLIMB), Inc.

P.O. Box 91377

Anchorage AK 99509

Phone: 907-222-5321

Email: climb@pobox.alaska.net (Jean Kollantai)

❖ www.FirstCandle.org

First Candle/SIDS Alliance is a nonprofit health organization uniting parents, caregivers and researchers nationwide with government, business and community service groups to advance infant health and survival.

First Candle/SIDS Alliance

1314 Bedford Avenue, Suite 210

Baltimore, MD   21208

Phone: 1-800-221-7437

Email info@firstcandle.org.

❖ www.Hygeia.org

The Hygeia Foundation, Inc. & Institute for Perinatal Loss and Bereavement is an organization whose mission is to comfort those who grieve the loss of a pregnancy or newborn child, to address disparities in access to healthcare services for medically and economically underserved families with respect, dignity and advocacy and to provide advocacy and resources for maternal and child health.

Hygeia Foundation, Inc.
PO Box 3943
New Haven, Connecticut, 06525 USA
Phone: 1-800-893-9198 Fax: 1-800-893-9198
Email: berman@hygeia.org

❖ www.MarchofDimes.com
The March of Dimes is an organization whose mission is to improve the health of babies by preventing birth defects, premature birth, and infant mortality.

March of Dimes
1275 Mamaroneck Avenue
White Plains, NY 10605
Phone: 914-428-7100

❖ www.MISSChildren.org
The MISS Foundation (Mothers in Sympathy and Support) is a volunteer-based organization committed to providing crisis support and long term aid to families after the death of a child from any cause. MISS also participates in legislative and advocacy issues, community engagement and volunteerism, and culturally competent, multidisciplinary, education opportunities.

MISS Foundation
P.O. Box 5333
Peoria, Arizona, 85385
Phone: 623-979-1000   Fax-1-623-979-1001

❖ www.MissingGRACE.org
The Missing GRACE Organization helps families on their journey through pregnancy and infant loss, infertility and adoption. They provide support and resources to aid individuals as they Grieve, Restore, Arise, Commemorate and Educate; and commit to make available educational opportunities that will help bring about awareness and prevention of stillbirth.

The Missing GRACE Organization
P.O. Box 1625
Maple Grove, MN 55311
Phone: 763-497-0709

❖ www.MyForeverChild.com
Unique keepsakes, jewelry and gifts to comfort those touched by the loss of
a child, no matter what age—miscarriage, stillbirth, pregnancy loss, newborn baby, infant, older child and adult loss.

Susan Mosquera
P.O. Box 541
East Northport, NY 11731
Phone: 1-888-325-2828

❖ www.NationalShareOffice.com
The mission of Share Pregnancy and Infant Loss Support, Inc. is to serve
those whose lives are touched by the tragic death of a baby through early
pregnancy loss, stillbirth, or in the first few months of life.

National Share Office
St. Joseph Health Center
300 First Capitol Drive
St. Charles, MO 63301-2893
Phone: 1-800-821-6819 or 636-947-6164   Fax: 636-947-7486
Email: share@nationalshareoffice.com

❖ www.ncjwny.org
The National Council of Jewish Women, New York Section, Perinatal Loss
and Support Program (PLSP) offers nationwide telephone counseling and
support groups in the New York metropolitan area to those who have experienced miscarriage, stillbirth or newborn death as well as to those who are
pregnant after a loss.

NCJW New York Section
820 Second Avenue
New York, New York 10017-4504
Phone: 212-687-5030   Fax: 212-687-5032
Email: info@ncjwny.org

❖ www.October15th.com
Remembering Our Babies works with local, state and national leaders to obtain a National Day of Remembrance recognizing the need for community education and awareness when a family loses a child to miscarriage, stillbirth, and/or neonatal death.

Robyn Bear
Remembering Our Babies
3210 Ewing Drive
Manvel, TX. 77578
Phone: 381-770-4553
Email robyn@october15th.com
Personal Website http://www.pain-heartache-hope.com

❖ www.PLIDA.org
The Pregnancy Loss and Infant Death Alliance, or PLIDA, is a nationwide, collective community of parents and health care professionals. We work together to ensure that all families experiencing the death of a baby during pregnancy, birth, or infancy will receive comprehensive and compassionate care from diagnosis through the reproductive years.

PLIDA
P.O. Box 658
Parker, CO 80134
1-888-546-2828, then press 3.
Email info@plida.org

❖ www.PostPartum.net

Postpartum Support International's website is intended only to increase knowledge on postpartum issues.

Postpartum Support International
927 N. Kellogg Avenue
Santa Barbara, CA 93111
Phone: 805-967-7636   Fax: 805-967-0608
Email: PSIOffice@earthlink.net

❖ Pregnancy and Infant Loss Center (no website available)
1421 East Wayzata Blvd., #30
Wayzata, MN 55391
Phone: (612) 473-9372; Fax: 612-473-8978

PILC provides referrals, literature, educational programs, volunteer opportunities, and many publications, including a newsletter, "Loving Arms," and the handbook, *Empty Arms.*

❖ www.Sidelines.org
Sidelines National Support Network is a non-profit organization providing support, education, advocacy and resources to women and their families during a high risk or complicated pregnancy or premature birth.

Phone: 1-888-447-4754

❖ www.StillbirthAlliance.org
The International Stillbirth Alliance (ISA), a non-profit coalition of organizations founded by stillbirth parents, is dedicated to understanding the causes and prevention of stillbirth.

International Stillbirth Alliance
1314 Bedford Avenue, Suite 210
Baltimore, MD 21208

❖ www.StillNoMore.org   The mission of the parent-led National Stillbirth Society is to "educate, agitate and legislate" for greater stillbirth awareness, research and reform.

National Stillbirth Society

P.O. Box 10273

Phoenix, AZ 85064

Phone 602-216-6600

Email stillnomore@cox.net

❖ www.Thumbies.com

Designers of fingerprint keepsake jewelry.

Meadow Hill Co., Inc.

405 Midway Street

Fox River Grove, IL 60021-1204

Phone: 1-877-THUMBIES (848-6243)/1-847-462 - 0701

Fax: 1-847-462 - 0703

❖ www.WintergreenPress.com

The Website of Sherokee Ilse-Bereaved Parent, International Speaker and Author of *Empty Arms* and many other books.

Wintergreen Press

3630 Eileen Street

Maple Plain, MN 55359

Telephone/Fax 952-476-1303

Email: SherokeeIlse@yahoo.com

Getting Off "Baby" Ad Lists

If you are getting "baby" junk mail and wish to get off the list write to:
Mailing Preference Service, P.O. Box 9008 Farmingdale, NY 11735.

For telephone solicitation removal:

Mailing Preference Service Phone Preference, P.O. Box 9014, Farmingdale, NY 11735.

This won't stop every call or mailing, but will catch the bulk and may take several weeks to take effect.